**Basic principles of
nuclear magnetic resonance imaging**

Basic principles of nuclear magnetic resonance imaging

J. Valk, M.D., Ph.D.,
C. MacLean, Ph.D. and
P.R. Algra, M.D.
Departments of Diagnostic Radiology and
  Chemistry
Free University
Amsterdam
The Netherlands

1985

Elsevier

Amsterdam - New York - Oxford

© 1985, Elsevier Science Publishers B.V. (Biomedical Division)

ISBN 0-444-80666-0

Published by:
Elsevier Science Publishers B.V.
(Biomedical Division)
P.O. Box 211
1000 AE Amsterdam
The Netherlands

Sole distributors for the USA and Canada:
Elsevier Science Publishing Company, Inc.
52 Vanderbilt Avenue
New York, NY 10017
USA

Library of Congress Cataloging in Publication Data

Valk, J.
  Basic principles of nuclear magnetic resonance imaging.

  Translation of: Inleiding in de Kernspin.
  Bibliografie: p.
  Includes index.
  1. Magnetic resonance imaging. I. MacLean, C.
II. Algra, P. R.   III. Title. [DNLM: 1. Nuclear Magnetic Resonance-diagnostic use.
WN 445 V174i]
RC78.7.N83V3513   1985   616.7'57   85-6903
ISBN 0-444-80666-0 (Elsevier Science Pub. Co.)

Printed in the Netherlands

Prologue

In 1946, Felix M. Bloch (Stanford University) and Edward M. Purcell (Harvard University) published independently their observations on Nuclear Magnetic Resonance, for which they were awarded the Nobel Prize for Physics in 1952. In 1973 nuclear magnetic resonance imaging (NMRI) began to develop, due mainly to the work of Paul C. Lauterbur (State University of New York), who introduced linear gradients for spatial resolution of NMR signals. /

A similar observation was made by Peter Mansfield (University of Nottingham). Many others have contributed to the further development of NMRI. To complete the picture, we should mention that Raymond Damadian, in 1972, applied for a patent on T_1 relaxation time measurements in the human body (published in 1974). Damadian did not use linear gradients but, nevertheless, was able to select a small, homogenous volume for his measurements (the so-called 'sensitive point' method). It is possible to construct images by moving an object point by point through this volume.

Because of existing CT scan experience with image reconstruction and the rapid development of minicomputers, NMRI was able to develop quickly. At the present time about 100 installations are working in clinical settings. It is evident that clinicians will be confronted more and more with this new imaging modality. This book tries to provide clinicians, radiologists and technicians who may become involved in NMRI with a basic understanding of this imaging process.

In CT scanning only one image per slice can be obtained. Image manipulation is only possible after digitalization of the absorption measurements (window and level setting, smoothing, edge enhancement, etc.) In NMRI, specific conditions for the image are set, with the choice of pulse sequence, pulse interval and pulse repetition time. One may alter these parameters to obtain images of different characters and containing different information. One

vi   image alone will not suffice to supply all the information available.

Therefore, it is obvious that the NMRI diagnostician must have knowledge of the basic physics of NMRI to be able to interpret the image correctly. This book is meant to help clinicians understand these basic NMRI principles.

Acknowledgements

We would like to express our gratitude to Technicare Corporation for their assistance in the preparation of this book, especially to Betty McAlpine and John C. Allen.

We are also deeply indebted to our secretaries, Lenie De Vries, Marion Meerwaldt, Anita Rijser and Inez Sloothaak, who have helped us through the many revisions. We thank E.W. Bastiaan for recording a number of NMR spectra.

Contents

Introduction

1

I. GENERAL

In this book the process of NMR imaging is analysed. Chapter 2 deals with the physics of NMRI, chapter 3 with the pulse sequences, chapter 4 with the localization of NMR signals in three dimensions, chapters 5 and 6 with the equipment. Chapter 7 deals with the clinical applications. The last chapters deal with spectrometry, contrast agents and biological hazards. First, however, we will discuss the place of NMRI in diagnostic procedures compared to other modern imaging modalities, i.e., computed tomography (CT), ultrasound (US) and digital subtraction angiography (DSA). Such an evaluation is only short-term since all these systems will continue to develop. The chapter on clinical applications is not a complete survey of all the work published to date. We intend to give only an impression of the clinical value of NMRI, illustrated by clinical state of the art images. A more complete survey of clinical applications of NMR will be presented in a separate volume.

II ULTRASOUND (US)

Ultrasound scanning, especially real-time scanning, is a diagnostic procedure which has gained great popularity because of the versatility and mobility of the system, the relatively low cost, the non-invasiveness and the biologically harmless radiation.

US images have improved considerably in the last 5 years. With the growing quality of the images, there is also a corresponding increase in price, though the equipment is still relatively cheap.

The spatial resolution is, as a rule, less than that of CT or NMR, and the image is degraded by gas in the bowels and the lungs. The adult skull is impermeable to US waves, unless there is an acoustic window following a surgical fenestration. In children with an open fontanelle excellent images of the cerebrum can be obtained (Figs. 1 and 2). In practice, US is the first choice for diagnosis of intracranial

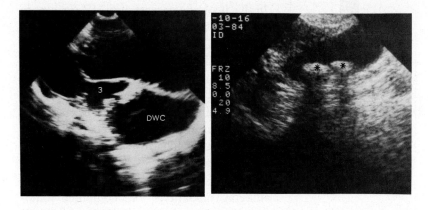

Figure 1. Ultrasound: transfontanelle sagittal real-time sector scan of a child with hydrocephalus and Dandy Walker malformation (fourth ventricle cyst).

Figure 2. US images of a gallbladder in which two stones (∗) are visible. The 'shadow' behind the stones is typical for this diagnosis.

lesions in new born children. It is also evident that in obstetrics and gynaecology US has become of great importance, because of its harmless nature. It is often used in initial examination of the upper abdomen (liver, gallbladder, spleen, pancreas) and of the kidneys, bladder and prostate gland.

US can also be used in radiological interventions, such as US-guided biopsies and US-guided drainage of hydronephrosis, abscesses, cysts, etc. Further developments will consolidate even more the already acknowledged position of US diagnosis as both a unique diagnostic tool and a screening device.

III DIGITAL SUBTRACTION ANGIOGRAPHY

The development of DSA has been quite different from that of US. In a very short time the potential of this diagnostic medium has been developed almost completely, and spectacular new advances should not be expected. From the point of view of diagnostic imaging, this method has offered nothing fundamentally new. By digitalization and storage of a series of fluoroscopic images in the memory of a computer, it has become possible to visualize the differences between two images, analogous to the principle of photographic subtraction as described long ago by Ziedses des Plantes. Digitalizing this process makes it possible to enhance the signals, so that the arteries are visualised clearly after intravenous injection of radiographic contrast material. Manipulation of the digital data is, of course, possible. Flow curves, estimations of the cardiac ejection fraction, etc., can be made. The established indications for DSA via the intravenous route are: disorders of the thoracic and abdominal aorta, the neck vessels, renal arteries, bifurcation of the abdominal aorta, pulmonary vessels and the lung parenchyma. This information is obtained by means of injecting relatively large quantities of contrast medium: e.g., 40 ml per projection. Often four or five series are necessary, totalling up to 200 ml of contrast medium (Fig. 3). For older patients, or patients suffering from cardiac or pulmonary dysfunction, renal insufficiency or diabetes, this is a large amount.

DSA is certainly not a safe alternative method of examining patients who would otherwise be considered at too high a risk for angiography. In these patients the examination is certainly invasive, even though it can be done on an outpatient basis. Apart from the examinations mentioned, DSA is of importance in the control and follow up of postoperative cases, especially after vascular surgery. Unfortunately, thus far it has not been possible to use the method as a

4

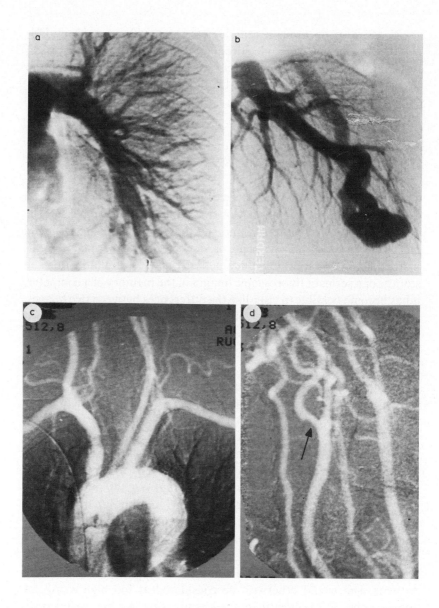

Figure 3. DSA. a. and b, Images of the pulmonary artery and its branches in a normal subject (a) and in a patient with an arterial-venous shunt (b). c and d, Analysis of the aortic arch and the neck vessels in a patient with transient ischaemic attacks (TIA). The aortic arch shows elongation (c); the right carotid artery shows an atheromatous lesion at the bifurcation (arrow).

test for patency of coronary bypasses. Improvement of the spatial resolution may eventually make it possible to use intravenous DSA for control studies of delicate surgical interventions, e.g., intracranial aneurysm clipping. The intra-arterial application of DSA has a great future and eventually will replace most conventional angiography. Instant subtraction images speed up the procedure, make it possible to reduce the amounts of injected contrast medium and allow the use of even smaller catheters. In interventional angiography, DSA also speeds up the procedure and allows better and immediate visualisation of results. However, application of DSA is restricted compared with that of US, CT and NMR. It will have a place of its own in medical imaging techniques.

IV CT SCANNING

In barely one decade CT has found a highly important place in diagnostic imaging, not only for the brain, as predicted in the early days, but for an ever growing number of areas in the body. Short scan times, highly increased spatial and density resolution and sophisticated software have all contributed to this success. Certainly, the possibilities of CT scanning have not yet been explored fully, and it is to be hoped that the enormous investment currently employed in the development of NMR will not be at the expense of further development of CT technology.

An important factor will be the differences in acquisition times: seconds per slice for CT, minutes per slice for NMRI. For NMRI of the thoracic and abdominal areas, gating, both respiratory and cardiac, is mandatory, which further lengthens the time of acquisition. Because of this, the throughput of patients on NMRI systems has been low: about four patients per day on resistive systems: six to eight patients per day on cryomagnetic systems. Probably NMR acquisition times will be shortened by improvement of software, contrast agents, pulse sequences, etc. However, the seconds/minutes ratio between CT and NMR will not change overnight in favour of NMRI (Fig. 4 a–f).

A second disadvantage of the NMR system as compared to CT is the difficulty in scanning patients with life-support and monitoring

6

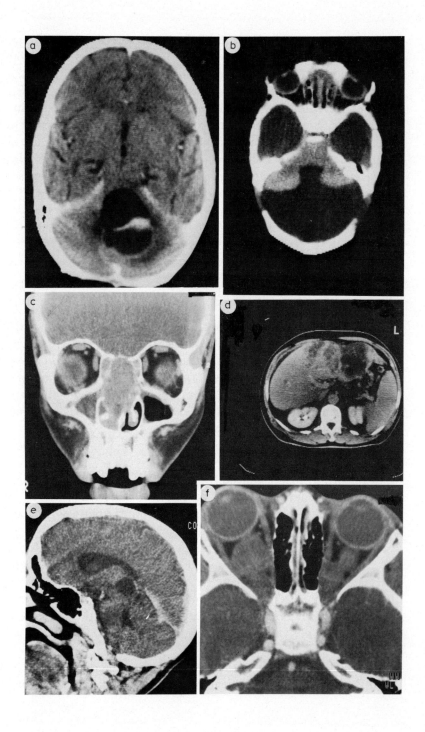

systems containing magnetic materials. At present, this means that for patients with acute trauma, patients depending on support systems and monitoring, premature babies, infants, patients who need sedation, etc., the CT scan will be the instrument of choice for both osseous and soft tissue diagnosis. This may seem to argue against NMR and in favour of CT, but that is not the point we are trying to make. It is despite these disadvantages that NMRI has already proven its clinical potential. The quality of information that can be obtained in soft tissue diagnosis is so different from CT scanning, and contains so much more important diagnostic information that we cannot permit ourselves to ignore the rapid development of this diagnostic modality.

What are the principal differences? In CT scanning the signal consists of the measurements per picture element of X-ray absorption by tissues. This measurement of the relative electron density of the tissue components is a passive phenomenon. By rotating the X-ray tube and the detectors around the object, projections in different directions are obtained, from which the image can be reconstructed. The densities, expressed as Hounsfield units, can be measured directly on the TV monitor on which the image is displayed. It is possible to change the slice thickness and the dose for better spatial resolution, but principally the signal contains the same information. Unfortunately, the differences in density are not specific enough to allow more accurate tissue characterization, e.g., differentiating malignant from benign tissue. Therefore, CT scanning will continue to be used primarily as a morphological examination, though some extra information may be gained by intravenous injection of radiographic contrast material, eventually enhancing differences in tissue by differentials in uptake, or testing the permeability of the blood-brain barrier.

Figure 4. Some of the possibilities of modern CT scan examinations. a, So-called 'trapped' fourth ventricle after treatment for a medulloblastoma in the posterior fossa. b, Dandy Walker cyst (compare US image in Figure 3). c, Tumour in the nasal cavity and occlusion of the right maxillary sinus. d, Lesion in the liver, probably primary gallbladder carcinoma. e, Direct sagittal image in child with hydrocephalus and cyst in the pineal region. f, Bilateral neurofibromas in the orbit. These and many other applications of CT have made this instrument the cornerstone of modern diagnostic radiology.

The NMR signal is of a completely different nature from that of CT. What the NMR image reconstructed from this signal will be like depends, amongst other things, on the choice of pulse sequence, gradient fields, and the strength and duration of radiofrequency transmission, which are all dictated by the examiner (chapter 3). The signal itself is a resonance signal generated by the nuclei of atoms in the human body.

In the present NMR imaging techniques the proton (^{1}H), the nucleus of the hydrogen atom, is the principal component. The H atom consists of a proton and an electron. The natural abundance is 99.98%. The human body contains about 65% water and, apart from the H_2O molecules, protons are present in other compounds linked to $C(H_2)$ and $N(H_2)$. Therefore, the conditions in the human body for proton imaging are almost ideal. The sensitivity of the proton for NMR is also high. The proton can be considered as a small, rotating sphere with an electric charge. A rotating or spinning charge has a magnetic field around it: the nucleus has a magnetic moment. In a macroscopic sample, and in the absence of a magnetic field, the magnetic moments of the nuclei are distributed equally in all directions. The net magnetic moment is zero. In a strong external magnetic field this situation changes: the protons align either parallel or antiparallel to the magnetic field and the summation of all these small magnetic moments leads to a relatively large magnetic moment, parallel to the main magnetic field. Radiofrequency pulses satisfying certain resonance conditions (chapter 2) can tip the magnetic vector away from this direction. Rotating around the magnetic field, the magnetic vector can induce a signal in a correctly placed 'receiver' coil. The signal strength is in the first instance proportional to the total number of nuclei present (protons in our case). The process of restoring the magnetic vector along the static magnetic field, after the RF pulse has ceased, is called relaxation. Relaxation times of tissue components are of great importance in NMRI (chapters 2 and 3). Their values are characteristic of the speed with which the equilibrium situation is restored following the RF pulse. Two relaxation times can be distinguished: T_1, or longitudinal, and T_2, or transverse relaxation time. Pulse sequences can be chosen in such a way that the image is dominated either by the proton density or by one or both of the relaxation times. In chapter 2 we will discuss this extensively. For the moment it is sufficient to realize that, unlike CT scanning, we are not dealing with only one NMR image, but that we have a number of choices. The image is the result of a number of selected parameters and also of the characteristics of the examined nuclei in the object. This opens up the possibility of tissue characterization, which has yet to be explored fully. At this moment differentiation of various kinds of tissues in the NMR image is often superior to that obtained by CT. In the head, where movement artefacts play a minor role, its superiority over CT has already been proven. In body imaging, NMR has to be performed with cardiac and/or respiratory gating. Our illustrations will demonstrate that when this is done the superiority of NMR over CT is apparent in clinically important 'whole body' areas, such as the mediastinum and the pelvis. The possibility of obtaining images in any desired plane is, in this respect, of great importance. For other organs US and CT are clearly competitive.

VI 'NUCLEAR' MAGNETIC RESONANCE IMAGING

In the USA and Great Britain, and latterly in other parts of Europe, there has been a tendency to change the name NMRI (nuclear magnetic resonance imaging) into MRI (magnetic resonance imaging). The motive for doing so is the supposed negative psychological impact of the word 'nuclear', because of its association with nuclear arms, warfare, waste, etc., which could deter people from using a valuable diagnostic tool. On the contrary, we are of the opinion that it is unwise to behave like the ostrich, and prefer to trust the ability of reader and patient to distinguish between bonafide and detrimental applications of scientific knowledge. Besides, the word 'nuclear' decribes exactly the kind of magnetic resonance that the method is based on, and distinguishes this form from other types of magnetic resonance.

Elementary considerations about NMR

2

I INTRODUCTION

In the condensed phases, liquids and solids, NMR was first observed by Felix Bloch (Stanford University) and Edward M. Purcell (Harvard University) in 1946. These observations confirmed a suggestion of the Dutch physicist C.J. Gorter in 1932, namely that when molecules or atoms are placed in a strong magnetic field, transitions can be induced between different nuclear spin states. Since about 1950 NMR spectroscopy has been an important device in investigations into the structure of organic and inorganic compounds. In modern chemical laboratories NMR spectrometers are an absolute necessity. In its simplest form an NMR spectrometer consists of a magnet, a radiation source, and a detector system, which measures the absorption of the radiation (Fig. 5). The sample is placed in the magnetic 'field' of the magnet.

In order to obtain NMR absorption, the nuclei of the atoms must have a 'magnetic moment'. In that case, the nuclei behave like elementary, small magnets. Not every atomic nucleus has this property. Table 1

12

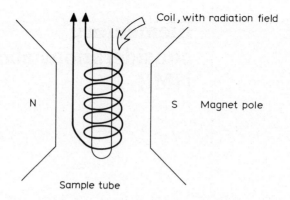

Figure 5. Schematic representation of an NMR spectrometer.

Table 1

Examples of nuclei with a magnetic moment

Atom	Symbol	Natural abundance	Spin quantum number, I	Gyromagnetic ratio
Hydrogen	^{1}H	99.98%	$\frac{1}{2}$	$2.6753 \cdot 10^8$ seconds^{-1} Tesla^{-1}
Deuterium	^{2}H	$9.65 \cdot 10^{-3}$	1	0.4107
Carbon (isotope: 13)	^{13}C	$1.59 \cdot 10^{-2}$	$\frac{1}{2}$	0.6728
Nitrogen (isotope: 14)	^{14}N	99.63	1	0.1934
Fluorine	^{19}F	100	$\frac{1}{2}$	2.5179
Sodium	^{23}Na	100	3/2	0.7081
Phosphor	^{31}P	100	$\frac{1}{2}$	1.0840

Examples of atomic nuclei without a magnetic moment are: ^{12}C, ^{16}O, ^{28}Si, ^{32}S and ^{40}Ca. The possible number of nuclear orientations in a magnetic field is not the same for all nuclei. It is two (parallel and antiparallel) in the case of ^{1}H, ^{13}C, ^{19}F, ^{31}P (and for many other nuclei), and three in the case of ^{2}H and ^{14}N: parallel, perpendicular and antiparallel. The number of possible orientations may exceed 10. In general we can say that the number of possible orientations is $(2I+1)$, where I is the spin quantum number. In the case of ^{1}H, $I = \frac{1}{2}$ and in the case of ^{2}H, $I = 1$, etc. The spin quantum number I characterizes the 'angular momentum' (thus, the mechanical moment) of the nucleus. Its magnitude is equal to: $\sqrt{I(I+1)}$ $(h/2\pi)$, where h is the Planck constant. γ is the ratio of the magnetic moment and the angular momentum. The resonance frequency of the nucleus can be calculated from: $\nu = (1/2\pi) \gamma H_0$, where ν is expressed in Hz and the magnetic field H_0 in Tesla, or expressed in the angular frequency $\omega = 2\pi\nu$ so that ω (seconds^{-1}) $= \gamma H_0$

shows some elements whose nuclei have magnetic moments. A good example is the nucleus of the hydrogen atom, the proton.

The nuclei of atoms with a magnetic moment can be regarded as small tops which spin around their axes (Fig. 6a). The charge of the nucleus also rotates, and the result is a rotating current which can be regarded as a small magnet. In an NMR experiment the nuclei are placed in a strong magnetic field. In such a field the elementary magnets align along the field direction, similar to a compass needle in the magnetic field of the earth. However, an important difference is that the magnetic moments of the atomic nuclei can only take a few discrete orientations in the magnetic fields. Protons only have two possible orientations, parallel and antiparallel (Fig. 6b). It will be evident that the parallel orientation has the lowest potential energy. In a given

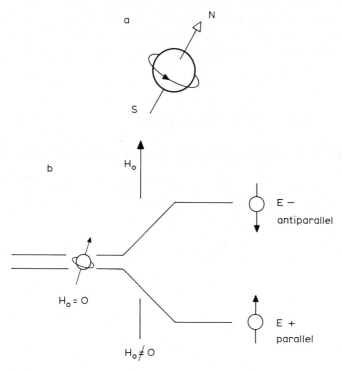

Figure 6. a, Model of a rotating or 'spinning' nucleus. b, When a proton is placed in a magnetic field, its magnetic moment can take only one of two orientations, either parallel or antiparallel to the magnetic field. The first orientation has lower potential energy than the second. In zero field, the levels coincide.

magnetic field, H_0, there is a constant energy difference between the parallel and the antiparallel orientation.

The radiation source (Fig. 1) induces transitions between the parallel and antiparallel orientations. It is clear that the frequency of the radiation field, ν, should correspond with the energy difference between the parallel and the antiparallel orientation, ΔE. According to a well known theory of quantum mechanics, the 'quantum' of the radiation, $h\nu$, has to be equal to the energy difference, ΔE:

$$\Delta E = h\nu \qquad\qquad\qquad\qquad (2.1.)$$

'h' is the Planck constant; its numerical value is $6.67 \cdot 10^{-34}$ Joule/second. In classical NMR spectrometers the radiation was applied continuously to the sample. In modern spectrometers the radiation is applied in 'pulses'. During one pulse a great number of oscillations of the radiation field take place. For the following discussion, it is not important how the radiation is applied, continuously or pulsed.

II   THE RESONANCE CONDITION

The potential energy of a magnetic dipole, placed in a magnetic field H_0, is given by

$$E = -\mu\, H_0 \cos \theta \,(\text{Fig. 7})$$

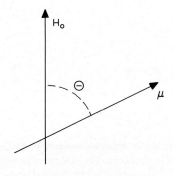

Figure 7. See text.

μ is the dipole moment of the magnetic dipole; it measures the magnitude of the dipole. θ is the angle between the directions of μ and H_0. The formula expresses that the potential energy is least when the dipole is parallel to the field ($\theta = 0$). In the case of an antiparallel orientation ($\theta = \pi$) the potential energy is maximal. The point zero is chosen at $\theta = \pi/2$.

The magnetic dipole moment of a nucleus of an atom is related to its angular momentum, the mechanical moment of the nucleus. To illustrate this, we can imagine an electron describing circular motion in a plane with constant velocity. The magnetic moment is equal to the product of the magnitude of the current and the area

$$\mu = iS = \nu e S$$

The current i is equal to the product of the frequency, ν, of the circular motion and the charge, e. If R is the radius, $S = \pi R^2$ and $\mu = \nu e \pi R^2$. The angular momentum, L, of the electron is equal to the product of the momentum mv (m, electron mass), and the radius of the circle R:L = mvR. Expressing the velocity, v, of the electron in the frequency ν by $v = 2 \pi R \nu$, gives the relation between the magnetic moment and the angular momentum:

$$\mu = \frac{e}{2m} L$$

For obvious reasons, the factor e/2m is called the 'gyromagnetic' ratio, usually indicated by the symbol γ. In this elementary system: $\gamma = (e/2m)$. By analogy, the magnetic moment of the nucleus of an atom is written as $\mu = \gamma L$. The gyromagnetic ratios of practically all magnetic nuclei are known. As an example, the gyromagnetic ratio of a proton is $2.6753 \cdot 10^8$ second $^{-1}$ Tesla $^{-1}$. Numerical values of γ of a number of nuclei are given in Table 1. The orientation energy of a nucleus in a magnetic field H_0 can now be expressed as

$$E = - \gamma H_0 L \cos \theta \qquad (2.2)$$

Angular momenta of atomic nuclei have only discrete values; they are expressed in units of Planck's constant, $h/2\pi$ (which has the dimension of angular momentum) and the so-called spin quantum number

'I', which is known for all nuclei (see, e.g., Table 1). The following relation holds:

$$L = \sqrt{I(I+1)} \, \frac{h}{2\pi}$$

For a hydrogen nucleus, $I = \frac{1}{2}$ and $L = \frac{1}{2} \sqrt{3} \, (h/2\pi)$ Joule/second; for a deuteron, $I = 1$, and $L = \sqrt{2} \, (h/2\pi)$. Now we express the orientation energy, E, as a function of the spin quantum number, I:

$$E = -\gamma \frac{h}{2\pi} \sqrt{I(I+1)} \, H_0 \cos \theta$$

Finally, we should know the possible orientations of a nuclear spin in a magnetic field. An abundance of experimental data reveals that $\cos \theta = (m / \sqrt{I(I+1)})$ where the 'magnetic quantum number', m, can have only $(2I+1)$ values: $m = I, I-1, \ldots, -(I-1), -I$. In the case of a proton $I = \frac{1}{2}$ and $m = +\frac{1}{2}, -\frac{1}{2}$. These values correspond with the parallel and antiparallel orientations. In the case of a deuteron, $I = 1$, so that $m = 1, 0, -1$. There are three orientational possibilities: parallel, perpendicular and antiparallel in relation to the magnetic field. The orientation energy is thus given by $E = -m \gamma (h/2\pi) H_0$, in which $m = I, I-1 \ldots, -I$. In the case of a proton the orientational energies are $E_+ = -\frac{1}{2} \gamma (h/2\pi) H_0$ and $E_- = +\frac{1}{2} \gamma (h/2\pi) H_0$.

In Figure 8 the energies are drawn as a function of the field. The energy difference between the two possible orientations is given by:

$$\Delta E = E_- - E_+ = \gamma \frac{h}{2\pi} H_0 \tag{2.3}$$

With equation 2.1 we can find the relation between the radiation frequency, ν, and the field, H_0

$$\nu = \frac{1}{2\pi} \gamma H_0 \tag{2.4}$$

This equation should be considered as a 'resonance condition': the protons can change their orientation if the frequency of the radiation

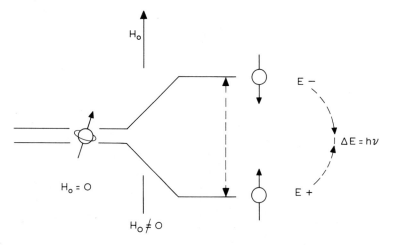

Figure 8. Orientation energies of a proton in a magnetic field H_0. At the left side $H_0 = 0$ and the levels coincide; on the right, both levels are drawn as a function of H_0. The longer vertical arrow represents the energy of the quanta of the radiation field. At the field value indicated by the arrow ΔE and and $h\nu$ fit each other and the resonance condition is satisfied.

and the magnitude of the magnetic field fit each other (Eqn. 2.4). If this is not the case, the radiation has little or no effect. In discussing this matter further, we assume that the strength of the magnetic field is 1 Tesla ($= 10,000$ Gauss); for proton NMR the required frequency of the radiation is 42.6 MHz. This frequency falls in the range of the so-called radio frequencies.

In the case of NMR with nuclei other than protons, the frequency of the radiation has a different value. For example, for ^{13}C NMR (in a field of 1 Tesla) the resonance frequency is 10 MHz. In the case of stronger magnetic fields the frequencies are proportionally higher. However, the quanta are always small in comparison with the quanta which are applied in diagnostic radiology. If we express the energy of the X-ray quanta in frequency units, the number is close to 10^9 MHz. The quanta used in NMR imaging are many orders of magnitude smaller in energy; at a low intensity they can be considered to be without danger for tissues.

To clarify further the previous discussion, Figure 9 depicts the NMR spectrum of the benzene molecule, C_6H_6, measured in the liquid phase. This molecule has six identical protons, which give rise to

18

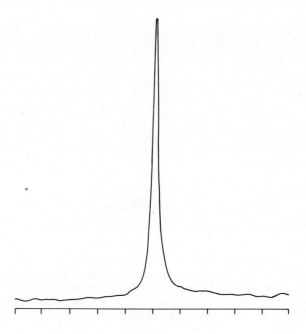

Figure 9. The proton spectrum of benzene consists of one line. In the figure the frequency of the radiation field is constant and the magnetic field varied, but of course this could be reversed: the field could be kept constant, with a variable frequency.

the NMR signal. Along the vertical axis, the intensity of the absorbed radiation from the radiation field is given, and horizontally the strength of the magnetic field. The position of the absorption line is dependent on the field strength, H_0, as expressed by Equation 2.4. The variation of the field H_0 in Figure 9 in fact takes place over a very small range. One should assume that in Figure 9 the constant field H_0 (for example 1 Tesla) is varied over a range of only $10^{-5} - 10^{-6}$ Tesla. Clearly, the line width of the NMR line is very small.

III THE CHEMICAL SHIFT

Soon after the first observations of NMR the chemical shift was discovered. Figure 10 shows the NMR spectrum of a mixture of benzene, nitromethane, cyclohexane and tetramethylsilane. Here, as in Figure 9, we deal with the NMR spectrum of the protons in the molecules. In

the first instance we might expect a single line in the spectrum, but we
see the four molecules separately. The peak intensities reflect the frac-
tions of the four compounds in the mixture. These shifts are explained
by a slight shielding of the field by the electrons in the molecule: the
magnetic field at the position of a proton is not exactly the same as the
externally applied field, but is somewhat smaller. If the magnetic field
at the nucleus is written as $H_0 (1 - \sigma)$, where σ is the chemical shift,
then the resonance condition (Eqn. 2.4) would become

$$\nu = \frac{1}{2\pi} \gamma H_0 (1 - \sigma) \qquad (2.5)$$

Because of the great resolution potential of NMR spectrometers, the
differences in Figure 10 seem considerable, while the chemical shifts
of protons vary only between 10^{-5} and 10^{-6}.

For convenience we usually express σ in 'parts per million' (ppm).
Experiments show that the chemical shift is proportional to the field;
this is also expressed by Equation 2.5. Although the chemical shift

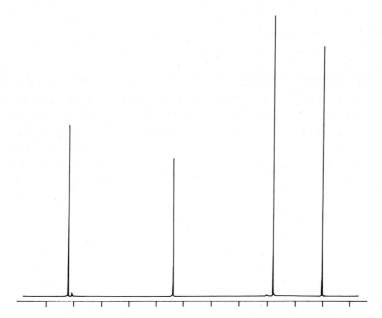

Figure 10. The proton NMR spectrum of a mixture of benzene (C_6H_6), nitromethane
(CH_3NO_2), cyclohexane (C_6H_{12}) and tetramethylsilane ($Si(CH_3)_4$).

plays an important role in the analysis of molecules, we do not have to consider this phenomenon in the case of NMR imaging. The NMR line widths of protons in the human body are so large that, unless the field of the spectrometer is very high, the chemical shifts cannot be seen separately. However, developments in this field are well on their way and separate images of the distribution of water and fat in tissue can already be made.

For indirect spin-spin couplings, discussed in the next section, no developments in the NMR imaging technique can be expected.

IV   THE INDIRECT COUPLINGS

In the preceding section, chemical shifts were considered. In practice, further splittings of the NMR lines are found. They are the result of the so-called indirect couplings. These phenomena can best be clarified by an example. Consider the molecule, ethanol: $HO-CH_2-CH_3$. There are three resonances in the NMR spectrum of the protons: of the OH group, the CH_2 group and CH_3 group (Fig. 11). These three resonances, of which the surface ratios are 1:2:3, reflect the differences in chemical shift of the three groups of protons. With a stronger magnetic field H_0, and thus with a higher frequency of the radiation field, ν, the distances between the resonances are proportionally greater. As the homogeneity of the magnetic field increases there are further splittings of the NMR lines (Fig. 12); the methylene group shows a quartet structure (intensities, 1:3:3:1) and the methyl group a triplet structure (1:2:1). The splittings of the lines are independent of the magnetic field, in contrast to the chemical shifts, which are proportional to the field. The reason for the multiplet structure is the existence of the already mentioned indirect spin-spin couplings. The distances between the different resonances shown in Figure 12 are very small: the distance between two components of the quartet of the CH_2 group is about $2 \cdot 10^{-7}$ Tesla, or about 8 Hz. In order to observe these small effects, which are independent of the field H_0, a high-resolution spectrometer is needed. Therefore, these spectra are known as high-resolution spectra. Just like chemical shifts, the indirect couplings are important in the analysis of the structure of molecules. However, they can be neglected in the case of NMR imaging of tissues. The reason is

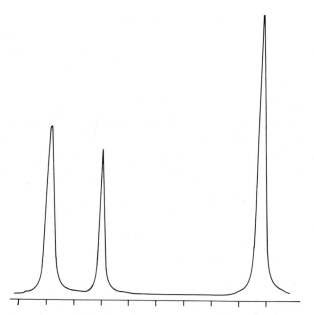

Figure 11. The proton NMR spectrum of ethanol with low resolution. Left to right: CH_2, OH and CH_3. For experimental purposes chloroform was added to the sample. Because of this, the OH resonance is shifted to a higher field strength. In pure alcohol the OH group falls at lower field.

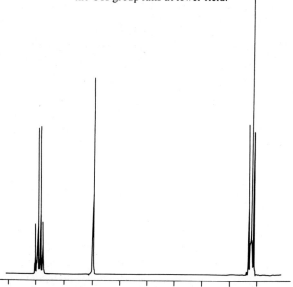

Figure 12. High-resolution proton NMR spectrum of ethyl alcohol, after addition of a small quantity of acid or base. In the case of pure alcohol, there would also be a splitting of the OH resonance.

obvious: the NMR lines of protons in tissue are relatively wide, because the mobility of the molecules is relatively low. High-resolution spectra can only be obtained in liquids with low viscosity. The latter can be illustrated by the NMR spectra of ice and water. On freezing, the width of the spectrum increases from, say 0.1 Hz, to a few thousand Hz.

As soon as Brownian motion is suppressed, the NMR lines become wider, as is clear from the example of ice (Fig. 13). In tissues and organs the 'thermal motion' is almost, but not completely, suppressed. As a result the spectrum is so broad that the fine structure of chemical shifts and indirect couplings cannot be measured. In the case of NMR imaging of tissue they can, for the time being, be ignored.

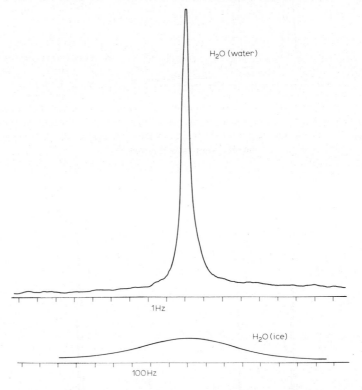

Figure 13. The NMR spectra of water and ice. Because of the Brownian motion the line width of water is small, about 0.1 Hz. Depending on the temperature, the spectral line of ice is broad, about 4000 Hz. The scales of the top and bottom figures differ by about 1/100.

An experimental concept of great importance in NMR imaging is 'relaxation' of nuclear spins. To illustrate this concept, the two energy levels of protons are shown in Figure 14: one corresponds to the parallel and the other to the antiparallel orientation with respect to the magnetic field. It is clear that in thermodynamic equilibrium the number of parallel protons should be larger than the number of antiparallel protons, because the energy of the former orientation is lower. In fact, there are two competing tendencies. From the standpoint of energy, it would be favourable if all protons were parallel to the field. However, temperature tends to equalize the two populations. The competition between the two tendencies results in an excess of protons with the parallel orientation, but the occupation difference is very small: for every million spins there are only a few more in the lower energy state than in the higher one. This small difference, however, is the base for the possibility of detecting NMR signals.

Imagine that a sample tube, filled with water, is placed at a certain

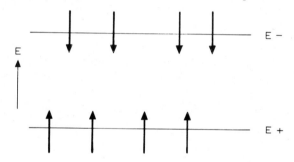

Figure 14. See text.

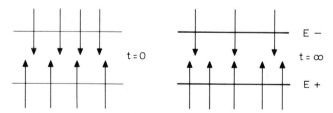

Figure 15. Distribution at t = 0 and at t = ∞ of the orientations of proton spins. A limited number of spins is drawn.

instant of time (t = 0) in a magnetic field. The protons first will be divided equally over both energy levels (Fig. 15). By means of relaxation processes, the equilibrium distribution will develop.

In Figure 16 the difference between the respective populations, n_+ and n_-, are drawn as a function of time. In practice, the equilibrium distribution is usually reached via exponential growth from zero to the final value. We first discuss the final value of $(n_+ - n_-)$. It is shown, in appendix 1, that in equilibrium the difference in population is proportional to the energy difference between the parallel and antiparallel orientation (ΔE) and inversely proportional to kT, the product of Boltzmann's constant and the absolute temperature

$$(n_+ - n_-) = \frac{N}{2} \left(\frac{\Delta E}{kT} \right) \tag{2.6}$$

N is the total number of protons in the sample. The quotient ($\Delta E/kT$) is small: for protons in a field of about 1 Tesla, ($\Delta E/kT$) is equal to $10^{-5} - 10^{-6}$. The curve in Figure 16 can be described mathematically by the formula:

$$(n_+ - n_-) = \frac{N}{2} \left(\frac{\Delta E}{kT} \right) (1 - e^{-t/T_1}) \tag{2.7}$$

After a long time, t, the exponential is negligible and the right side can

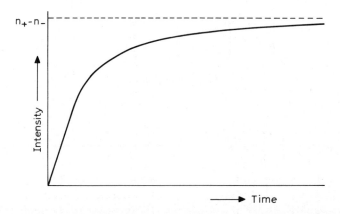

Figure 16. The growth of the difference between the respective populations n_+ and n_- as a function of time. The curve is represented by Equation 2.7. From this curve the relaxation time, T_1, can be calculated. For the protons in water, $T_1 \approx 1$ second.

be formulated as in Equation 2.6; for t = 0, thus $e^0 = 1$, the right part
of the formula is equal to zero: the occupation numbers n_+ and n_- are
equal. At high temperatures the population difference is almost zero.
In strong magnetic fields ΔE is relatively large; therefore, the population difference and the NMR signal increase. The constant T_1 in
Equation 2.7 is a so-called relaxation time. It is a measure of the rate at
which equilibrium is reached. For $t = T_1$, $(n_+ - n_-)$ has increased to
63% of the final value. A simple method of measuring T_1 is the following: after having placed the sample in the field of the NMR spectrometer, the growth of the NMR signal is observed as a function of time
(see Fig. 17).

It is clearly of interest to have an idea of the magnitude of relaxation
times T_1 as found in actual practice. Table 2 shows values of T_1 of a
few commonly used liquids, together with their viscosities at the same
temperature. It is interesting that with lower viscosity, T_1 has a larger
value. Viscous liquids, such as glycerol, have short relaxation times.
The relaxation time of protons in water at room temperature is close to
1 second. A simple physical explanation of relaxation can be found in
the fluctuating dipolar fields, caused by neighbouring protons, at the
site of a specific proton. These time-dependent fields can induce transitions between the energy levels, in a way analogous to the one
described for a radiofrequency field.

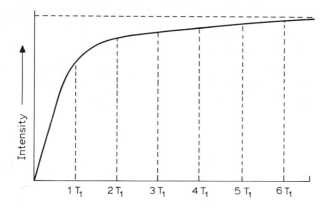

Figure 17. The growth of the NMR signals as a function of time. At time t = 0 (left in
the figure) the sample is placed in the field of the spectrometer. Via Equation 2.7, the
relaxation time, T_1, can be calculated from this curve.

Table 2

Proton relaxation times (T_1) of certain liquids

	Relaxation time (seconds)	Viscosity (cpoise)
Diethyl ether	3.8	0.25
Water	2.3	1.02
Ethyl alcohol	2.2	1.2
Acetic acid	2.4	1.2
Sulphuric acid	0.75	25
Glycerine	0.023	1000

Measured at 29 MHz and 20°C (adapted from: N. Bloembergen, dissertation, Leiden, 1948). Remark: In the case of molecules which have more than one type of proton (e.g., ethyl alcohol), T_1 has to be considered as the effective relaxation time of all protons. In fact, T_1 values can vary considerably within one molecule. In ethyl alcohol the protons of the CH_3, CH_2 and OH groups have different relaxation times (T_1).

In NMR imaging experiments the proton resonance of water in tissue and organs usually is measured. The effective viscosity of this partially bonded water would be considerable, and therefore the relaxation time, T_1, is short, for example, $10^{-3} - 10^{-4}$ seconds. According to the well-known theory of quantum mechanics, the spectral width of the transition involved has to be large. As a result, the differences in chemical shifts and indirect couplings cannot be observed in the spectra. To be specific: the line width of a spectral line and the life time of the energy levels involved are related by an 'uncertainty relation': if the life time of an energy level is short the energy level is not well defined and the spectral line is broadened. Theory predicts that the product of life time of the levels and uncertainty in transition frequency should be about 1. Or simply: a short life time of the levels involved will be characterized by a broad spectral line. Above, the short life time of the energy levels is caused by rapid relaxation. These considerations can explain the relatively large widths of NMR lines of water molecules in tissue.

In experiments it is often practical to consider the magnetic moments
of a population of nuclear spins instead of a single one. This is due to
the fact that the description of the behaviour of the net magnetic
moment of the population in static and radiofrequency fields is relatively simple. If we limit ourselves to macroscopic magnetic moments
we can, up to a certain level, even ignore the quantum mechanical
character of the nuclear spins. This means that classical mechanics
can be applied to explain the behaviour of the spin system. The total
magnetic moment of N nuclei, N being, for instance, Avogadro's number ($N = 6 \cdot 10^{23}$), is called the magnetization. It is the vectorial sum
of all magnetic moments in the sample and is designated by the symbol
$\vec{M}$. For some borderline situations the magnitude of M can be indicated without difficulty. For example, consider a sample of water in a
region where the magnetic field is zero. The direction of the magnetic
moment of the individual nuclei would then be randomly distributed
and the net magnetization is zero: $M = 0$. If all the nuclear spins are
parallel to each other, we have another borderline case. This situation
can only be created at extremely low temperatures. For the magnetization we can write: $M = N\mu$, where μ is the magnetic moment of one
nuclear spin and N is the number of spins. At normal temperatures,
even for the strongest magnetic field, the population difference
between parallel and antiparallel orientations of a spin system with
spin quantum number $I = \frac{1}{2}$ is small

$$(n_+ - n_-) \cong \frac{N}{2} 10^{-5}$$

(see the discussion of Equation 2.6). In the general case we could
write

$$M = (n_+ - n_-)\mu \tag{2.8}$$

where again μ is the magnetic moment of one nuclear spin. It will be
evident that $\vec{M}$ is a vector which in equilibrium is parallel to the existing magnetic field. Its length can be expressed by the equation above.
For the following discussion it is important to write the magnetization,
and thus the product $(n_+ - n_-)\mu$, in the following fundamental quan-

tities: N, the total number of nuclear spins; H_0, the magnitude of the static magnetic field; and γ, the gyromagnetic ratio. We consider first the factor $(n_+ - n_-)$ in Equation 2.8. We have already discussed (Eqn. 2.6) that the population difference of the energy levels of the nuclear spins can be written as $(N/2)\,(\Delta E/kT)$, where ΔE is the energy difference between the parallel and antiparallel orientations. If the strength of the magnetic field and the temperature are known, ΔE, and therefore $(n_+ - n_-)$, can be calculated easily. The second factor on the right in Equation 2.8 is the magnetic moment of one nucleus, or rather, the component of the magnetic moment of that nucleus along the direction of the applied magnetic field. In one of the previous paragraphs it was made clear that the two possible energies are: $\pm\,\tfrac{1}{2}\,\gamma\,(h/2\pi)\,H_0$. The minus sign stands for the parallel orientation and the plus sign for the antiparallel one. This situation can be also described as one where the magnetic field of the nucleus precesses around the magnetic field H_0 in such a way that its component along H_0 is constant in time and has the value of $\pm\,\tfrac{1}{2}\gamma\,(h/2\pi)$ (see Fig. 18).

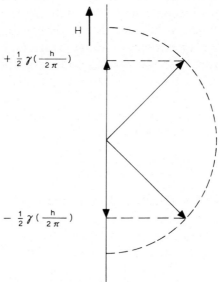

Figure 18. Quantum mechanical image of the two possible orientations of the magnetic moment of a proton in a magnetic field H_0. The oblique arrows represent the magnetic moment. The projections along H_0 can only have the values of $\pm\,\tfrac{1}{2}\,\gamma\,(h/2\pi)$. Therefore, the indications 'parallel' and 'antiparallel' should not be taken literally.

Substituting the above results, we find that the magnetization has
the magnitude

$$M = \frac{N}{2} \left(\frac{\Delta E}{KT}\right) \cdot \left(\frac{1}{2} \gamma \frac{h}{2\pi}\right) \tag{2.9}$$

With Equation 2.3, $\Delta E = \gamma (h/2\pi) H_0$, we finally arrive at

$$M = N \left(\gamma \frac{h}{2\pi}\right)^2 \frac{H_0}{4kT}$$

Therefore, a strong magnetic field produces a large magnetization, as could be expected intuitively. Furthermore, M is proportional to N, the number of protons in the sample. The dependence on temperature is also understandable: at high temperatures the difference in population $(n_+ - n_-)$ is small, as is the magnetization. In equilibrium, the direction of M is the same as the direction of H_0. Thus, with known magnitude of the field strength and the temperature, M is defined, in both direction and magnitude. In the following discussion it is important to understand that, in equilibrium, no magnetization perpendicular to the field exists. Evidently, there can be no preferential direction perpendicular to the field. If we conceive a coordinate system with H_0 parallel to the z-axis (Fig. 12), we can distinguish three components of the magnetization, M_x, M_y, and M_z. In equilibrium they have the magnitudes: $M_x = M_y = 0$ (Fig. 19);

$$M_z = N \left(\gamma \frac{h}{2\pi}\right)^2 \frac{H_0}{4kT}$$

In non-equilibrium situations, for instance after a radiofrequency (RF) pulse, M_x and M_y can differ from zero. The component of the magnetization along the z-axis, M_z, is also referred to as 'longitudinal' magnetization; therefore, the symbol M_l is also used often. M_x and M_y are components of the transverse magnetization, also indicated as M_{tr}. As mentioned before, in equilibrium only M_z differs from zero. However, it is possible to manipulate the spin system, e.g., with radiofrequency pulses, and to induce a tranverse magnetization. Of course, the system is then not in an equilibrium state. If left to itself the transverse magnetization will decay with a time constant called the transverse relaxation time, for which the symbol 'T_2' is used (see Fig. 20).

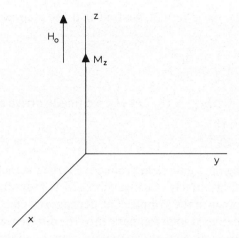

Figure 19. In thermodynamic equilibrium the magnetization is parallel to the field (in the figure, along the z-axis). In the directions perpendicular to the z-axis there is no magnetization: $M_x = M_y = 0$.

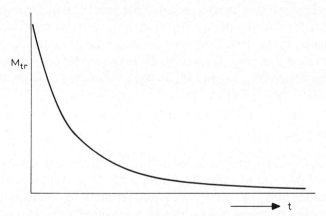

Figure 20. With a pulse at time $t = 0$ a transverse magnetization is produced, which decays in accordance with the equation $M_{tr} = M_i\ ^{-t/T_2}$. The time constant T_2 is the 'transverse' relaxation time. M_i is the initial value of the transverse magnetization.

VII   THE TRANSVERSE RELAXATION TIME

In the previous section the transverse relaxation time T_2 was introduced. It is obvious that the question arises of how much the numerical value of T_2 of a sample differs from the already discussed longitudinal relaxation time, T_1. In solids T_2 is usually much shorter than T_1. The difference can be of the order of 10^4–10^5. In liquids with low viscosity T_1 and T_2 generally are identical. In tissues and organs we have to do with an intermediate situation: T_2 is shorter than T_1, but not to the same extent as in solids. An important question is also: how can T_2 be measured? A possible way of measuring T_1 was already discussed previously. In the case of T_2, the situation is somewhat more complicated. We have to discuss first the concepts 'Larmor precession' and 'Larmor frequency'.

VIII LARMOR PRECESSION AND LARMOR FREQUENCY

In thermodynamic equilibrium the macroscopic magnetization, M, is aligned parallel to the magnetic field. By applying a radiofrequency pulse it is possible to bring the magnetization under an arbitrary angle, θ, with the magnetic field (Fig. 21). This leads to a transverse magnetization M_{tr} with magnitude $M \sin \theta$; the longitudinal magnetization has decreased after the pulse and has the magnitude $M_1 = M \cos \theta$. The total value of magnetization is unchanged: $M_1^2 + M_{tr}^2 = M^2(\sin^2 \theta + \cos^2 \theta) = M^2$. Suppose that after the pulse the spin system is left to itself. For the moment we disregard relaxation processes and follow the behaviour of M_1 and M_{tr} in time.

According to a theorem of Larmor (see Appendix 3) the magnetization M precesses around the field in such a way that M_1 is constant. M describes a cone with a constant angle θ; M and thus its projection on the transverse (x, y) plane precess around the magnetic field with the so-called Larmor frequency: ω_L (Fig. 22). The numerical value of ω_L is equal to the product of γ, the gyromagnetic ratio, and the static magnetic field, H_0:

$$\omega_L \text{ (second}^{-1}) = \gamma H_0 \tag{2.10}$$

or

$$\nu \text{ (Hz)} = \frac{1}{2\pi} \gamma H_0 \tag{2.11}$$

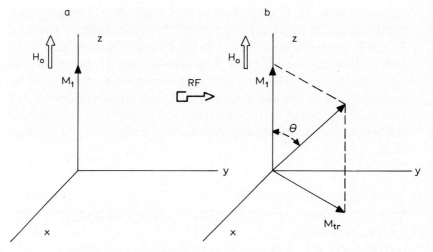

Figure 21. a, Before the pulse the spin system is in equilibrium and the magnetization is parallel to the field. b, After the RF pulse the magnetization makes an angle θ with the field.

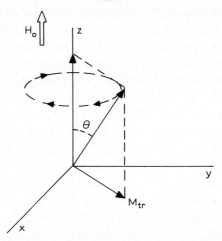

Figure 22. After the pulse the magnetization makes an angle θ with the field. The magnetization precesses around the field with the Larmor frequency.

In a field of 1 Tesla (10,000 Gauss) the Larmor frequency for protons is 42.6 MHz. It should be noted that the classical Larmor frequency from Equation 2.11 concurs with the quantum mechanical transition frequency (Eqn. 2.4) between the two stationary energy levels of a nuclear spin in a magnetic field.

In this discussion the relaxation processes have been omitted. After
a time, T_2, the transverse magnetization has largely decayed. Mean-
while, the longitudinal magnetization has increased and in time will
reach its equilibrium value (see Fig. 36).

In actual practice, both T_1 and T_2 are relatively long compared to
one period of the Larmor precession; hence, many precessions have
taken place before the longitudinal and transverse magnetizations
have decayed.

In Figure 23, assume that a coil is placed along the x-axis of the
frame. The coil is fixed in space and is crossed by the transverse magnetization, M_{tr}, with a frequency identical to the Larmor frequency.
An alternating voltage is induced in the coil, the amplitude of which is
proportional to the actual value of M_{tr}. Immediately after the pulse,
M_{tr} and thus the alternating current are maximal; after T_2 seconds the
amplitude has decreased to e^{-1} of its initial value, according to the
equation (see Fig. 13)

$$M_{tr} = M_i\, e^{-t/T_2} \qquad\qquad (2.12)$$

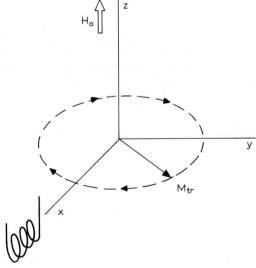

Figure 23. The precessing transverse magnetization induces an alternating voltage in
the receiver coil. The longitudinal magnetization cannot be observed directly with the
coil.

The time constant T_2 is the transverse relaxation time; the transverse magnetization at time t = 0 has the value M_i.

From the previous discussion a simple method can be derived to measure T_2: the alternating voltage induced in the receiving coil can be plotted against time. From the change in amplitude as a function of time, T_2 can be obtained (Fig. 24). The described phenomenon is called the 'free induction decay' (FID) and the measured alternating voltage the 'free induction signal'. In experiments the measurement of T_2 will be influenced by the inhomogeneity of the magnetic field H_0 (Fig. 35). The Larmor frequency $\omega_L = \gamma H_0$ will not be the same over the whole sample. This leads to a small, but not unimportant, spread of the resonance frequencies. The decay of the transverse magnetization will be mainly dependent on these small differences. How T_2 can be measured with exclusion of the contributions of the field inhomogeneities will be discussed later.

IX THE ROTATING FRAME

As we have seen, it is possible to manipulate the magnetization by means of a radiofrequency pulse: the magnetization (see Fig. 21) can be turned into any desired direction. We will now describe this phenomenon more accurately.

In an NMR spectrometer the sample is submitted to a strong static magnetic field, H_0, and a weak radiofrequency field, H_1. If only H_0 is present, M aligns along the direction of H_0. If M is turned away from

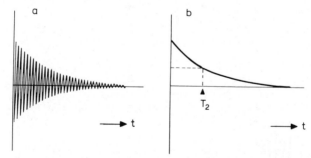

Figure 24. a, At time t = 0 a transverse magnetization is produced with an RF pulse. A periodic alternating voltage is induced over the ends of the receiver coil with the Larmor frequency ω_L. The amplitude decays according to Equation 2.12. b, After detection of the alternating current an exponentially decaying curve is measured, allowing direct measurement of T_2.

this orientation by a radiofrequency pulse, the magnetization precesses around H_0 with the Larmor frequency $\omega_L = \gamma H_0$, in such a way that the longitudinal component of M, M_l, is constant (Fig. 22). The weak alternating RF field, H_1, is perpendicular to the static field, H_0. It is produced by a coil, the transmitter coil, in which a current flows, generated by an oscillator. The direction of H_1, of course, coincides with the axis of the transmitter coil: the RF magnetic field is 'polarized' along the coil axis. This alternating field can be assumed to be composed of two fields rotating in opposite directions (Fig. 25). One of these components rotates in the same direction as the Larmor precession, the other rotates in the opposite direction. Because the latter has no effect on the magnetization, it can be neglected. Though the RF field is polarized along the axis of the coil, only one component of the rotating field H_1 has to be taken into account (see Appendix 3). The frequency of the RF field, ω, will as a rule be close to the Larmor frequency ω_L, but is not necessarily identical to it.

Apart from the laboratory frame of reference (x,y,z) we can now introduce a frame (x', y', z') that rotates with the RF field. Because

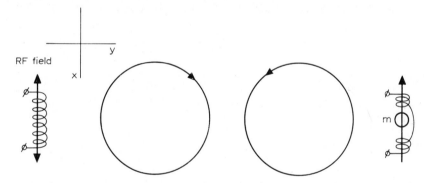

Figure 25. In NMR spectrometers the RF field is generated by a 'transmitter' coil, through which an alternating current flows. It is placed perpendicular to the static magnetic field, H_0 (see also Fig. 5). The RF field lies along the axis of the coil, and thus is a linear field. However, this RF field can be conceived as the superposition of two RF fields, rotating in opposite directions. The component rotating against the Larmor precession can be neglected, because it has no effect on the magnetization. In Figure 23 the 'receiver' coil has already been introduced. Often transmitter and receiver coil are identical. The dimensions of transmitter coils vary, from about 1 cm in NMR spectrometers to 50 cm or more in whole-body NMR imaging equipment. 'Surface coils' are often used as receiver coils (see Ch. 5); their dimensions are adapted to those of the tissue under investigation. m, sample tube.

the RF field lies perpendicular to H_0, the z- and z'-axes are parallel. Let us now consider which magnetic field is observed in the rotating frame (x',y',z') (see Fig. 26).

In the first place, the RF field in the rotating frame (x',y',z') will be seen as a static field. It is more difficult to understand how the static field H_0 is experienced in the rotating frame. In Appendix 4 it is demonstrated that the apparent static field is smaller (or larger) than H_0, the difference depending on the RF frequency, ω. By applying the correct radiofrequency the static magnetic field H_0 can even become zero. it can be shown (see Appendix 4) that in the rotating frame the field along the z'-axis can be written as $(H_0 - (\omega/\gamma))$. Notice that (ω/γ) has the dimension of a magnetic field. If ω, the frequency of the RF field, is identical to ω_L, the Larmor frequency, no static field is present in the rotating frame; only H_1 is present. In Figure 27 these various situations are presented graphically.

The behaviour of the magnetization in a constant field has already been discussed previously: M precesses around the static field in such a way that the component of M along the field remains constant in time. We now refer to the situation in Figure 27b, where $\omega = \omega_L$. The RF field is exactly in resonance, and in the rotating frame only H_1 is present and constant in time. Therefore, the magnetization will precess

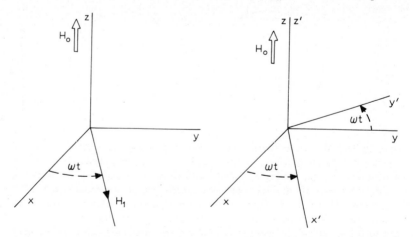

Figure 26. On the left the laboratory frame of reference is represented. The RF field rotates in this frame with the frequency ω. The rotating frame, on the right, rotates with the H_1 field. In this frame H_1 is a constant vector (which precesses with regard to the laboratory frame with the angular velocity ω).

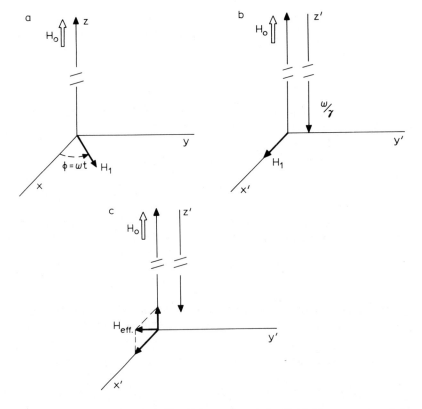

Figure 27. a, In the laboratory (fixed) frame (x,y,z) the RF field rotates around the direction of H_0 with the frequency ω. In this frame H_1 is seen under a time-dependent angle, $\phi = \omega t$, with the x-axis. b, The rotating frame (x',y',z'), rotating with the RF field, is now introduced: H_1 is chosen along the x'-axis. Contrary to Figure 27a, H_1 is now a static vector. Introduction of the rotating frame leads to a change of the static field H_0 along the z'-axis: $H_z' = (H_0 - (\omega/\gamma))$. If $\omega = \gamma H_0$, i.e., if the frequency of the RF field is identical to the Larmor frequency, the field along the z'-axis disappears. In the rotating frame the field H_1 now is the only field and it is, besides, constant in time. c, If ω is slightly different from the Larmor frequency there is a field $(H_0 - (\omega/\gamma))$ along the z'-axis and a field H_1 along the x-axis. The 'effective' field, H_{eff}, is the vectorial sum of these two fields. If $\omega = \omega_L$, $H_{eff} = H_1$, in accordance with the situation in Figure 27b.

around the x'-axis, the axis to which H_1 is parallel (Fig. 28). The precession frequency is $\omega_1 = \gamma H_1$, as is shown in Appendix 4. Because $H_1 \ll H_0$ also $\omega_1 \ll \omega_L$: during one precession around H_1 many precessions have taken place around H_0. The behaviour of the magne-

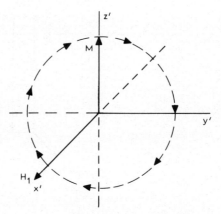

Figure 28. At resonance, $\omega = \omega_L$, the static field H_0 is cancelled by (ω/γ) and H_1 is the only field in the rotating frame. In equilibrium M is parallel to the z'-axis. As soon as H_1 is turned on, M starts to process around the static field H_1 with frequency $\omega_1 = \gamma H_1$. Relaxation processes are not considered; this approximation is allowed if the relaxation times are long, relative to the time of one precession.

tization, as observed in the laboratory frame (x,y,z), is represented in Figure 29. The magnetization precesses rapidly around H_0 and slowly in the direction of the negative z'-axis. By applying the RF field for a short time only, in other words by applying an RF pulse, it is possible to

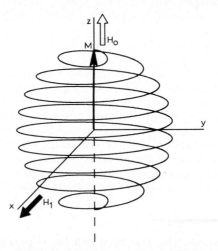

Figure 29. The precession shown in Figure 28, but now displayed in the laboratory frame. The slow precession around H_1 is superimposed on the fast precession around H_0.

bring the magnetization under a certain angle θ with the field H_0. If θ
= 90° we speak of a 90° pulse, if θ = 180° of a 180° pulse, etc.

X   THE 90°, 180° PULSE CONCEPTS

In thermodynamic equilibrium the magnetization M is parallel to the
static magnetic field, H_0. In NMR it is often important to bring M in a
direction perpendicular to H_0. This can be effected with a 90° pulse.
The RF field H_1 is turned on time t = 0. If $\omega = \omega_L$ the magnetization
M will start to rotate uniformly around the field H_1 with frequency ω_1
= γH_1. The angle θ between M and the z-axis is a function of time; we
can write $\theta = \omega_1 t$, in which t is the length of the pulse. In the case of a
90° pulse $\theta = (\pi/2)$ and the length of the pulse can be described as

$$t = \frac{\pi}{2} \cdot \frac{1}{\omega_1} = \frac{\pi}{2} \cdot \frac{1}{\gamma H_1} \tag{2.13}$$

If, after t seconds, the field H_1 is turned off the magnetization will just
have arrived in the transverse plane. Immediately after the pulse the
free induction decay (FID) is measured, as was explained earlier.
From Equation 2.13 we can infer that a strong RF field H_1 goes
together with a short pulse. If $H_1 = 10^{-4}$ Tesla we find, after substitution of γ, a pulse length of 30 μseconds. Generating pulses of this
length is a simple matter. It is obvious that the length of a 180° pulse
will be twice that of a 90° pulse. After a 180° pulse the magnetization
is directed antiparallel to the static magnetic field H_0 (Fig. 30). Clearly, the angle θ can be chosen at will by a correct choice of the length of
the pulse.

XI   MEASUREMENT OF T_1 OF A SAMPLE

The discussion in the previous section serves to introduce a commonly
used method to determine T_1. A spin system in equilibrium is submitted to a 180° pulse. Immediately after the pulse the magnetization is
directed antiparallel to the static magnetic field. The restoration of the
magnetization as a function of time is presented graphically in Figure
31.

After the pulse, thermodynamic equilibrium is disturbed and relaxation processes come into action to restore equilibrium. After a 180° pulse no transverse magnetization exists. The longitudinal magnetization, will, via the value zero, increase until the equilibrium value is

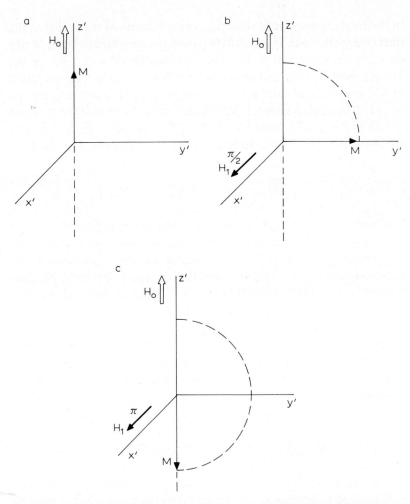

Figure 30. In the rotating frame the field H_1 has a time-independent direction in the transverse plane, e.g., along the x′-axis. a, In thermodynamic equilibrium the magnetization M is parallel to the field H_0, along the positive z′-axis ($H_1 = 0$). b, After a 90° pulse M is nutated into the transverse plane. c, After a 180° pulse M is parallel to the negative z′-axis, and therefore antiparallel to H_0.

restored (see Fig. 31). The characteristic time in which the final value is reached is the already discussed longitudinal relaxation time T_1 (see Fig. 16). We have seen previously that for the detection of an NMR signal a transverse magnetization is required; only the transverse magnetization can induce an alternating voltage over the ends of the receiver coil (Fig. 23). In practice, this problem is solved by applying a 90° pulse to the actual longitudinal magnetization, M_l, bringing it in the transverse plane. The amplitude of the FID measured immediately after the pulse is proportional to M_l. By varying the pulse interval time between the 180° pulse and the 90° pulse in successive experiments, M_l can be measured as a function of time and T_1 obtained. The experiment is depicted schematically in Figure 32.

In the foregoing we have assumed that $\omega = \omega_L$, and therefore that the resonance condition is satisfied, as illustrated in Figure 27b. When ω and ω_L are slightly different the precession will not take place around the field H_1, but around the effective field H_{eff}. In a sample there will always be some spread of the resonance frequencies, for example because of the chemical shifts of the spins. This would mean that the angle θ varies somewhat over the sample. However, this can be

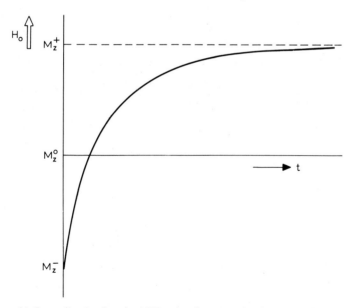

Figure 31. Immediately after the 180° pulse the magnetization is parallel to the negative z'-axis. The curve indicates the value of the magnetization as a function of time.

42 circumvented by choosing an RF field of sufficient strength. From Figure 27c we read

$$H_{eff} = \sqrt{H_1^2 + (H_0 - \frac{\omega}{\gamma})^2}$$

$$= H_1 \sqrt{1 + (H_0 - \frac{\omega}{\gamma})^2 H_1^2}$$

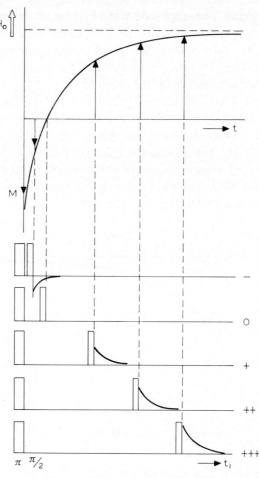

Figure 32. Measurement of the longitudinal relaxation time T_1. The sequence π - τ - $\pi/2$ (π indicating the 180° pulse, τ the interpulse time and $\pi/2$ the 90° pulse) is repeated a number of times for different times τ. The free induction decay (FID) is measured at a constant interval after the 90° pulse (as soon as the receiver has recovered from the pulse).

If the fraction under the root sign is small with regard to 1, then H_{eff} is practically identical to H_1 and the difference between ω and ω_L can be neglected.

XII SPIN ECHOES

Under conditions of thermodynamic equilibrium, in which the magnetization is parallel to the field H_0, the spin system is submitted to a 90° pulse. After a certain time, τ, a second 180° pulse is given, with $\tau \ll T_1$. After a time $2\,\tau$ a 'spin echo' is measured (Fig. 33). The spin echo phenomenon can best be explained with reference to the rotating frame. We assume that the RF field is along the x'-axis. Before the 90° pulse M is parallel to the z'-axis, the direction of the static magnetic field, H_0. Immediately after the 90° pulse M lies along the y'-axis; the longitudinal magnetization has been transformed into a transverse magnetization. This transverse magnetization will decay exponentially with a time constant T_2. During the decay the free precession signal is induced in the receiver coil, as shown in Figure 33. It is now important to take into consideration that the magnetic field over the sample is never perfectly homogeneous; this means that there exists a spread of Larmor frequencies. In some parts of the sample the Larmor frequency is somewhat higher, in other parts somewhat lower than the mean frequency. The microscopic magnetizations that add up to the net (macroscopic) magnetization do not stay aligned; they dephase. This can be visualized by looking at the transverse magnetization from a position along the z'-axis (Fig. 34).

Starting with the situation as given in Figure 34b we consider the influence of a 180° pulse on the transverse magnetization. This pulse will mirror all vectors with regard to the x'-axis, the direction of the RF field H_1. Both the slower and the faster precessing microscopic magnetizations proceed in the direction they already had. After a certain time all the microscopic magnetizations are again in phase and induce in the receiver coil the spin echo signal (Fig. 34).

The microscopic magnetizations can be considered as a group of runners which run with constant but different speeds. They start at the same time, but because of the differences in speed the cohesion in the group is lost. After a time τ a whistle is blown (180° pulse) and all the

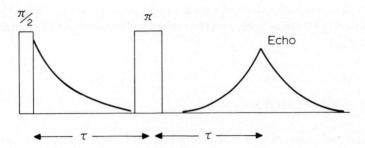

Figure 33. τ seconds after a 90° pulse the spin system is submitted to a 180° pulse. After 2τ seconds, a 'spin echo' appears. The condition $\tau \ll T_1$ implies that the growth of the longitudinal magnetization during the experiment can be neglected. This condition is well satisfied with, for instance, $T_1 = 1$ second and $\tau = 1$ msecond. In the imaging nomenclature τ is referred to as t_i; $2\,t_i = t_e$ (see also Nomenclature, section XVII).

runners start to run in the opposite direction, not changing their speed. After 2τ seconds they are all back where they started.

It will be obvious that a spin echo can be conceived as consisting of two FIDs, positioned back-to-back. Spin echoes can also be generated by other pulse sequences. We will not discuss the numerous variations.

XIII   MEASUREMENT OF T_2

The decay of the transverse magnetization is characterized by the time constant T_2. We have already discussed in the above section the influence of the inhomogeneity of the static magnetic field: the decay of the transverse magnetization occurs faster with worse homogeneity of the static magnetic field. In many instances, it is important to know the 'real' T_2, in which the influence of the field inhomogeneity is absent. To eliminate this influence the following method can be used: in successive experiments the amplitude of the spin echo is measured as a function of the parameter, τ, the interval between the 90° and the 180° pulses (Fig. 35). The echo amplitude, as a function of the inter-pulse time, τ, produces an exponential curve, from which the real T_2 can be calculated. The inhomogeneity of the magnetic field does not influence this experimental decay. This correction of field inhomogen-

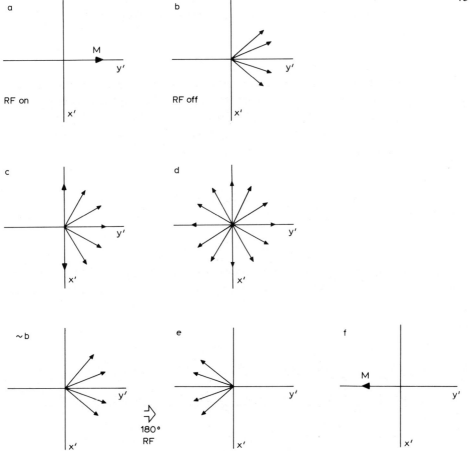

Figure 34. a, Immediately after the 90° pulse the magnetization (M) lies along the y'-axis of the rotating frame. b, c, Because of the inhomogeneities in the static field, H_0, the microscopic magnetizations dephase. If the local field is somewhat higher (lower) than the mean value the microscopic magnetizations are ahead (behind) in phase. d, Eventually the phases become distributed at random and $M_{tr} = 0$. The signal induced in the receiver coil is zero. e, Departing from the situation in Figure 34b, all the microscopic magnetizations are mirrored by a 180° pulse. f, After a time, 2τ, all microscopic magnetizations are in phase again and a spin echo is detected. Of course, the same reasoning applies if we start with the situation in Figure 34c.

eities is also used in other imaging pulse sequences. It should also be kept in mind that the T_1 and T_2 relaxation processes occur simultaneously (Fig. 36).

In the previous discussion it was assumed that there is no molecular diffusion during the measurement; however, if a molecule changes its place by diffusion during the measurement, the local field may change a little, and with it the Larmor frequency. These diffusion phenomena can usually be neglected in NMR imaging. In flow-measurements, for instance of blood flow, these diffusion processes are of paramount importance.

XIV   MEASUREMENTS IN THE DOMAINS OF TIME AND FREQUENCY

Spectroscopic measurements are usually presented in terms of wavelength or frequency of the applied radiation; in general, the absorption or the transmission of electromagnetic waves is plotted against either

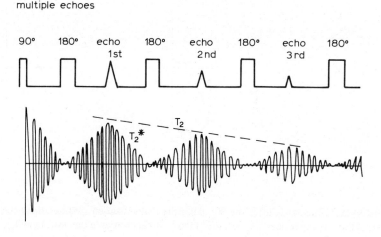

Figure 35. Graphic representation of the spin echo sequence and measurement of T_2. The measured T_2^* of the sample, as obtained from the free induction decay, decays faster than corresponds with the real T_2. To obtain the real T_2, a $\pi/2 - \tau - \pi$ pulse sequence is applied and a spin echo is generated. The amplitude of the spin echo decreases if the delay time τ is increased. From a plot of the echo amplitude versus t, the real T_2 can be inferred.

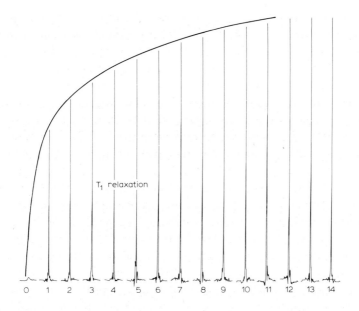

T₁ relaxation

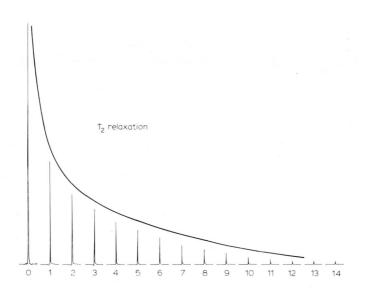

T₂ relaxation

Figure 36. Authentic T_1 and T_2 (longitudinal and transverse) relaxation measurements. The exponential relaxation curves are theoretical curves. Both relaxation processes occur simultaneously; in this example T_2 is shorter than T_1.

the wavelength or the frequency of the radiation. In electronic spectra (ultraviolet spectra or spectra in the visible range), the frequencies are of the order of 10^{14}–10^{15} Hz; vibration spectra of molecules are observed at frequencies of 10^{13}–10^{14} Hz, rotation spectra at 10^{11}–10^{12} Hz. The transition frequencies of NMR spectra depend on the field strength according to the relation $\nu = (1/2\pi)\gamma H_0$; at 1 Tesla the transition frequency for protons is about 42.6 MHz. In NMR spectrometers of the first generation, spectra were measured by scanning the magnetic field, keeping the RF frequency constant. In state of the art NMR spectroscopy the RF field is applied to the sample in short, intense pulses. The response of the spin system is the free induction decay (FID) (Fig. 24a) and the signal apparently is measured in the time domain. If we want to know the absorbed frequencies it is necessary to employ the so-called Fourier transformation, which transforms the time domain response to a frequency spectrum. In Figures 81 and 82 (Ch. 4) the relation between NMR signals, measured in the time and frequency domains, is sketched for a few specific cases. The conversion of a time domain signal to a frequency spectrum, i.e., the Fourier transformation of the time domain signal, is performed in practice by a computer. In present-day equipment, extensive Fourier transformations can be handled in short times, e.g., in a few seconds. For a discussion of the mathematical aspects of the Fourier transformation, the reader is referred to mathematical textbooks (see also Appendix 6).

XV ENCODING NMR SIGNALS IN TERMS OF POSITION

NMR imaging requires a procedure to encode the NMR signal of a specific volume element of the sample in terms of its position. This subject is treated in some detail in chapter 4. Here, we only mention the principle of the method which is currently in use.

The position of a piece of tissue of which the proton NMR is measured is fixed by way of the resonance condition $\omega = \gamma H_0$. The field H_0 is not constant from place to place: with linear gradients the field is made dependent on location. By use of the appropriate field gradients in three mutually perpendicular directions, a volume element (voxel) in the examined object can be identified. The NMR signals are always measured in the time domain and have to be converted to a frequency spectrum by a Fourier transformation.

XVI   SIGNAL AVERAGING

To obtain a good signal-noise ratio the RF pulse sequence is repeated a number of times. The free induction decay or the spin echo signal is stored after each pulse sequence in a multichannel analyzer, i.e., a memory with a number of channels. In a specific channel the amplitude of the FID or the echo at a well-defined instant of time is stored. All channels together contain the signal, split up in time increments. By repeating the pulse sequence the signal strength increases proportionally to the number of repetitions; contrarywise, the noise increases only with the square root of the number of pulse sequences (see Fig. 37). This fact is the principal reason to practice pulsed NMR: if N pulse sequences are used the signal to noise ratio (S/N) increases with $\sqrt{N}$. In principle, one could also repeat the measurement of the spectrum in the frequency domain N times; however, this would be very time consuming, as the spectrum has to be run through slowly to avoid broadening of the lines.

XVII   NOMENCLATURE

To indicate the different periods of time of the NMR pulse sequences, in this book the nomenclature is used as proposed by the American Society of Radiology, with one graphic difference. To avoid confusion we use small characters and subscripts instead of capitals (t_e instead of TE). In a pulse sequence we distinguish the initial pulse from the other pulses of the sequence. The final pulse in a sequence is the 'read pulse', after which the signal is collected in the memory of a computer. The time between two consecutive pulse sequences is indicated as t_r, pulse repetition time (in the references often denoted T_r or TR).

In the inversion recovery sequence (π-τ-($\pi/2$)), the ($\pi/2$) pulse can be regarded as the read pulse. The time τ between the initial pulse and the read pulse, τ, is indicated as t_i (T_i or TI); the subscript i refers to 'interpulse' time. In the spin echo sequence the spin echo time is usual-

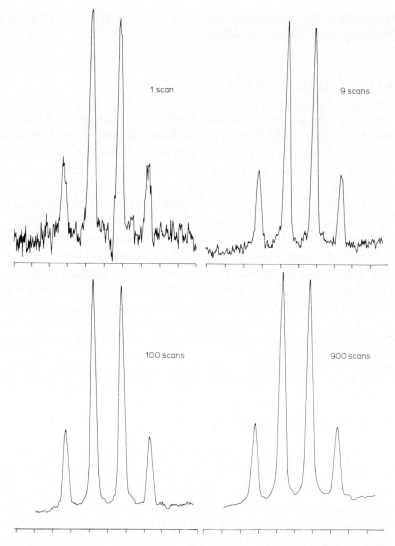

Figure 37. Effect of signal averaging on the S/N. With an increasing number of scans the noise decreases relative to the signal.

ly denoted by t_e (T_e or TE), twice the length of the time between the initial 90° pulse and the refocussing 180° pulse, which can be regarded as the read pulse ($t_e = 2t_i$). In a schematical representation of an inversion recovery sequence and, in fact, of all pulse sequences,

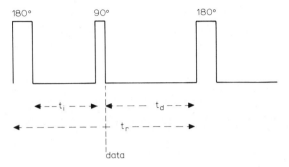

Figure 38. See text.

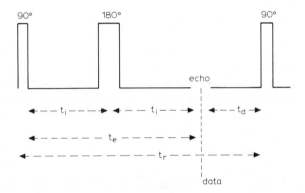

Figure 39. See text.

one time period still has to be indicated, i.e., the time between the read pulse and the next pulse sequence (see Fig. 38).

Though objections can be made against the name 'delay time', we will refer to this interval as t_d (T_d or TD). Given these indications, it is now possible to write the pulse sequences in shorthand

$$IR = \underbrace{(180° - t_i - 90° - t_d)}_{t_r} \underbrace{(180° - t_i - 90° - t_d)}_{t_r}, \text{ etc.}$$

The spin echo sequence can be drawn schematically as in Figure 39. Alternatively, we can write it as

$$SE = 90° - t_i - 180° - t_i - E - t_d \;\text{—}\!\!\text{—}|$$

$$\overset{\longleftarrow\qquad t_e \qquad\longrightarrow}{}$$

$$\overset{\longleftarrow\qquad\qquad t_r \qquad\qquad\longrightarrow}{}$$

Or, with multiple echoes,

$$MSE = 90° - t_i - 180° - t_i - E^1 - t_i - 180° - t_i - E^2 -, \text{etc.}$$

$$\overset{\longleftarrow\quad t_e \quad\longrightarrow \longleftarrow\quad t_e \quad\longrightarrow \longleftarrow}{}$$

first echo   second echo

$$\overset{\longleftarrow\qquad\qquad t_r \qquad\qquad // \text{—}}{}$$

In the set up of the pulse sequences t_d has no direct relevance; t_d is the delay time as a consequence of choosing the parameters t_r and t_i; in the inversion recovery sequence, $t_r - t_i = t_d$. Apart from the possibility of manipulating spin systems with different pulse sequences, saturation recovery (SR), inversion recovery (IR) and spin echo (SE), the NMR image can also be manipulated actively by the choice of t_i and t_r, as will be explained in chapter 3. It may be useful to reread this section after those chapters.

In the first chapters of this book, and in some of the equations, we have not followed completely the indications proposed here. For instance, τ is used instead of t_i, as is customary in NMR spectroscopy.

The pulse sequences in NMR imaging

3

I INTRODUCTION

The behaviour of magnetization with respect to static magnetic fields and RF fields was dealt with in the previous chapter. The generation of the NMR signal and the measurement of T_1 and T_2 were also discussed. In NMRI the difference in relaxation times of tissue components is most important, because it is responsible for the contrast in the NMR images. The differences in relaxation times will be seen as contrast in the NMR image in such a way that contrast is enhanced as the difference in relaxation times increases. Contrast can also be manipulated by the choice of specific pulse sequences. The principal pulse sequences are: saturation recovery (SR), inversion recovery (IR) and spin echo (SE). Nearly all other sequences currently used in NMRI are derived from these 'basic' sequences.

II SATURATION RECOVERY

One could say that pulse sequences, as used in NMRI, are, in a way, all saturation recovery sequences. However, it is customary to describe the 'FID' or 'repeated FID' pulse sequence as SR. This sequence can be schematically represented as follows:

$$\vdash 90° - t_d \longrightarrow \Vdash 90° - t_d \longrightarrow$$
$$\xleftarrow{\qquad} t_r \xrightarrow{\qquad} \xleftarrow{\qquad} t_r \xrightarrow{\qquad}$$

After the 90° pulse the precessing magnetization vector is oriented in the transverse plane, perpendicular to the z-axis (see Fig. 40). Immediately after the pulse, the amplitude of the recorded signal is proportional to the proton concentration of the studied sample. By means of this method a proton-density weighted image is obtained. Because of the strong signal emitted a favourable signal to noise ratio (S/N) can be obtained. However, there is little difference in proton density between the various tissues. For example, there is a difference of approximately 10% in water content between grey and white matter. Therefore, the SR image shows well-defined anatomical borders but limited differentiation of tissues. The differences in T_1 and T_2 are much more appropriate in discriminating various tissue components. A slight difference in water concentration may be responsible for a large T_1 difference (40–50 mseconds/1%). In order to highlight the T_1 differences in the tissues we have to change the SR pulse sequence, as will now be discussed.

Immediately after the 90° pulse, the z component of magnetization (M_z) is zero. Thereafter, the magnetization will return along the z-axis in an exponential way. This growth of M along the z-axis is characterized by the formula:

$$M_z = M_o (1 - e^{-t_i/T_1})$$

in which t_i is the interpulse time.
Substituting $t_i = T_1$ and with e = 2.71

$$M_z = M_o (1 - e^{-1}) \quad \text{or} \quad M_z = M_o (1 - \frac{1}{e})$$

$$M_z = M_o (1 - 0.37) \quad M_z = 0.63 \, M_o$$

This means that 63% of the original magnetization is restored when t_i

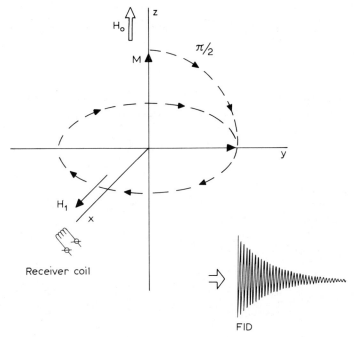

Figure 40. See text; the free induction signal is induced in the receiver coil by the component of the precessing M vector in the transverse plane.

$= T_1$. A graph representing the restoration of M_z to its equilibrium value is given in Figure 41.

For the measurement of the return of the magnetization along the z-axis it is necessary to apply once more a 90° pulse (Fig. 42). The amplitude of the subsequent FID is dependent on the speed of return of M_z, and therefore, especially with shorter t_i times, strongly dependent on T_1 (Fig. 43). With longer t_i times the amplitudes of the FIDs become less and less dependent on the T_1 times of the various tissue components and more and more dependent on the proton density. Therefore, in a SR sequence with $t_r > 5\,T_1$ the image will only display the proton density of the tissue.

It will be clear that to obtain T_1 weighted images we have to change the simple SR sequence. There are two methods to obtain T_1 weighted images:

1. After the initial 90° pulse a second 90° pulse is applied t_i mseconds later. Schematically:

56

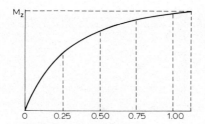

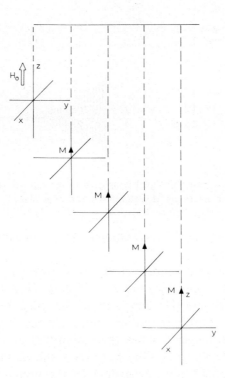

Figure 41. Relaxation following a 90° pulse. The magnetization tends to resume its original value in a process characterized by the relaxation time T_1. In the meantime, there will be transverse relaxation in the xy plane. Because of inhomogeneities of the H_o field and specific transverse relaxation processes, it will be completed earlier than the T_1 relaxation.

$$\vdash\!\!-90° - t_i - 90° - t_d -\!\!\vdash\!\!\vdash\!\! - 90° - t_i - 90° - t_d -\!\!\dashv$$

$$\vdash\!\!\!-\!\!\!-\!\!\!-\!\!\!- t_r -\!\!\!-\!\!\!-\!\!\vdash\!\!\!\!\!\mid_{\text{data}}\!\!\vdash\!\!\vdash\!\!\!-\!\!\!-\!\!\!- t_r -\!\!\!-\!\!\vdash\!\!\!\!\!\mid_{\text{data}}\!\!\dashv$$

The FID is recorded after the second 90° pulse. In Figure 42 the difference is shown between the signal amplitude after a short waiting time (t_i1) and a long waiting time (t_i2).

2. It is also possible to shorten the pulse repetition time (t_r). It will be evident that with a short repetition time ($t_r \ll 5\,T_1$), the magnetization along the z-axis will not have recovered its equilibrium value; for tissues with a longer T_1 relatively less than for tissues with a shorter T_1. Therefore, differences in T_1 between tissue components can also be accentuated by adapting the t_r. Figure 44 graphically represents a series of SR pulse sequences with short t_r.

Because there is no basic difference between the two sequences, we will restrict our discussion to the first sequence mentioned, collecting the data after having chosen an optimal t_i. In Figure 45 the T_1 relaxation of two different tissues is given, tissue 1 has a short T_1 and tissue 2 has a long T_1. The differences in restoration of magnetization with

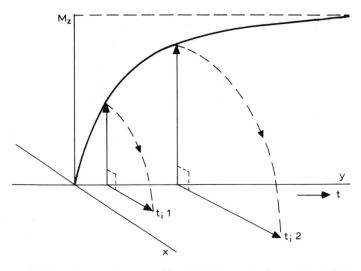

Figure 42. If one chooses a longer waiting time (longer t_i), the amplitude of the signal increases (n.b., to simplify the diagram the x-axis is turned to the right).

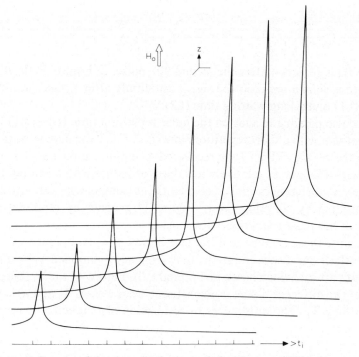

Figure 43. Increase of signal amplitude obtained after the second 90° pulse at various t_i times. The magnetization exponentially resumes its original value. In this example the intensity of a spectral line has been plotted as a function of time.

time are shown at two different interpulse intervals, t_i1 and t_i2. At the time t_i1, this difference has reached a maximum. The contrast plot for the interface between the two tissue components 1 and 2 is given in Figure 46.

For normal tissues, the T_1 and T_2 times, which are also dependent on the field strength, are well known. Contrast optimalization by a correct choice of interpulse (t_i) and pulse repetition (t_r) time is possible. The T_1 and T_2 times of pathological tissue in an actual examination are, of course, unknown: the abnormal tissue may have shorter (rarely) or longer (often) relaxation times than normal tissue. This point is most important in IR and SE sequences, where contrast inversions can occur (the 'cross-overs'). At the cross-over point the contrast is zero!

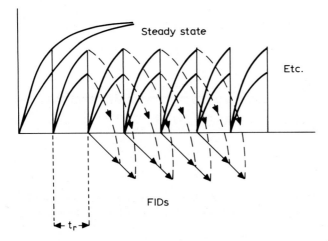

Figure 44. Schematic representation of the SR sequence with $t_r \ll 5\,T_1$. After each 90° pulse the signal amplitude is measured. Differences in T_1 of various tissues are emphasized; the signal intensity is less. This can be compensated for eventually by the possibility of having more scans in the same time. 'Steady state' refers to the practice of not making measurements before a 'stable' situation has developed.

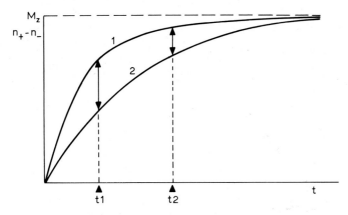

Figure 45. Curves for longitudinal relaxation of two tissues. Tissue 1 has a short T_1 and tissue 2 a long T_1. The difference is maximal (= maximal contrast) at t_i1.

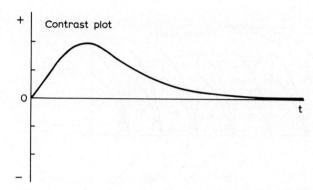

Figure 46. Contrast curve for the interface of the two tissue components in Figure 45, demonstrating an optimal t_i where the contrast is maximal.

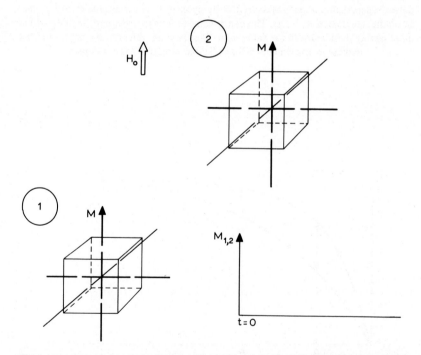

Figure 47. Also see text. Diagrammatic representation of two voxels containing different kinds of tissue with identical proton density. The M vectors along the z-axis are also identical. At time $= 0$ we have represented graphically (lower right) $M_z 1$ and $M_z 2$ in a state of equilibrium.

For the SR sequence the most efficient procedure is to shorten t_r.   61
Saturation pulses and read pulses are then identical. The T_1 differences of the tissue components are proportional to those obtained with
a sequence in which $t_r > 5\ T_1$ and with a separate 90° pulse applied
after t_i mseconds in order to obtain the data. The lower signal intensity
can be compensated for by the application of more pulse sequence
repetitions (signal averaging).

Let us consider what happens if two voxels (volume image elements) of the object under examination are placed in a static magnetic
field H_o. The initial position is represented in Figure 47. We assume
that the two voxels contain different kinds of tissue with about the
same amount of water (= proton density). The magnetizations of
voxel 1 and are, in this equilibrium state, identical: $M_z 1 = M_z 2$.

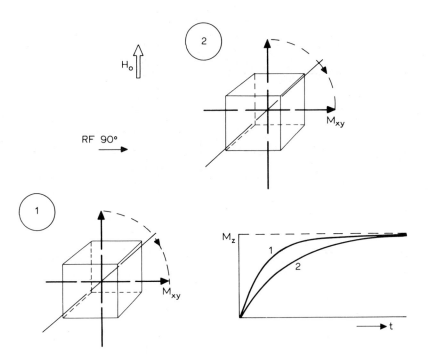

Figure 48. A 90° pulse has nutated the magnetization into the transverse plane. At time
$t = 0$, $M_z = 0$. The magnetization will return exponentially along the z-axis, with the
time constant T_1. For the tissues in voxel 1 and 2 these T_1 times are different, as shown in
the graph: T_1 for the tissue in voxel 1 is shorter than the T_1 for the tissue in voxel 2.

Now a 90° RF pulse is applied, affecting only the layer to which both voxels belong. The magnetization is rotated into the transverse plane; immediately after the pulse $M_z 1$ and $M_z 2$ are zero. When the RF pulse ceases, the magnetization of the two voxels will return exponentially along the z-axis. This exponential restoration of magnetization is characterized by the T_1 relaxation times of the two tissue components, which are different in this example. The exponential curves for the two voxels are illustrated in Figure 48.

After a certain delay, the interpulse time t_i, a new 90° RF pulse is given and the data are collected. The contrast in the images is now dependent on the differences in the T_1 times of the tissue components (Fig. 49). Note that the measurements concern the average T_1 of the tissue contained within the voxel.

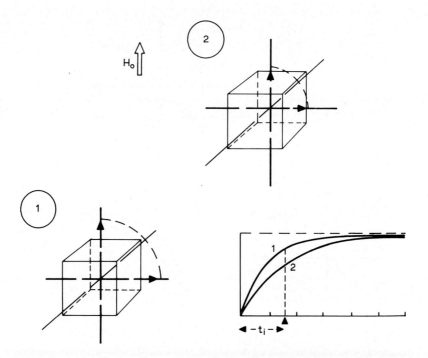

Figure 49. After a certain time, t_i, a measuring 90° RF pulse is applied. The contrast in the image is the result of the differences in relaxation, characterized by the relaxation times, T_1, of the tissue components.

With more voxels under consideration the same reasoning applies. The problem of locating the NMR signals in space is dealt with in chapter 4. The optimal t_i interpulse time, to obtain adequate contrast between tissue components, differs from organ to organ. In the brain this is in the order of 400 mseconds, in the kidneys closer to 200 mseconds. Often, however, the question arises of how to obtain optimal contrast difference between normal and pathological tissue. It sometimes is necessary to sacrifice the optimal contrast differences between healthy tissues in order to visualize the abnormal tissue.

It will be obvious that in the images obtained as described only relative values of the T_1 relaxation times are expressed in the images. The 'absolute' T_1 times (and in other sequences T_2 times) can also be measured and the calculated values expressed in a grey scale (= imaged). It is then necessary to measure the height of the relaxation curve (the signal intensity of the FID after the 90° RF pulse) for different t_i times. In practice T_1 is often calculated from measurements at two t_i times in the inversion recovery pulse sequence. The transverse relaxation time T_2 can be calculated from a spin echo sequence; T_1 and T_2 can be estimated roughly from the values obtained from an IR sequence with known t_i and a SE sequence with known t_e. As mentioned before, images can be reconstructed from the calculated T_1 and T_2 times.

III INVERSION RECOVERY

The contrast between the various tissue components can be enhanced by an initial pulse of 180° instead of 90°. After a 180° pulse the magnetization inverts along the z-axis, and immediately after the RF pulse is negative. After the pulse the magnetization returns exponentially or quasi-exponentially to the equilibrium situation in a period, characterized by the T_1 relaxation time (= longitudinal or spin-lattice relaxation time). In Figure 50 this recovery along the z-axis is represented schematically. The spin-spin (T_2) relaxation in the xy plane has been ignored in this representation.

The intensity-time curve for the return to equilibrium after a 180° pulse is shown in Figure 51 (see also Eqn. 2.11 and Fig. 31). In the first part of the curve (Fig. 51) the values of M_z are oriented along the

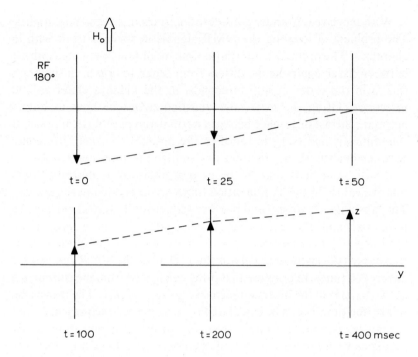

Figure 50. See text. Return of the magnetization along the z-axis after an initial 180°
pulse.

negative part of the z-axis. As in the SR sequence, the longitudinal
magnetization cannot be measured directly. It is necessary to give a
90° pulse to nutate the magnetization into the transverse plane, so that
an FID can be obtained (Fig. 52).

The contrast between two tissue components with a different T_1 is
dependent on both t_i and t_r. Similarly, in the SR sequence there is an
optimal t_i for maximum contrast between the tissues. However, the
contrast in the IR sequence is then twice that of the SR sequence. For
the brain this optimal t_i is about 400 mseconds (see Fig. 53). As was
already mentioned, the T_1 of pathological tissue is as a rule not known,
so that t_i cannot be set in advance for the best separation of normal and
pathological tissue.

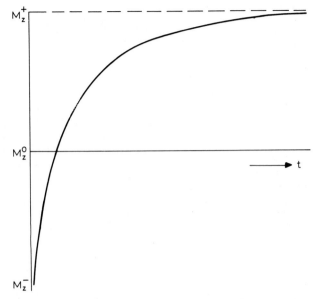

Figure 51. Schematic representation of the exponential increase of the magnetization in the inversion recovery sequence, according to the formula:

$$M_z = M_o (1 - 2 e^{-t_i/T_1})$$

The signal intensity, I, is dependent on the proton concentration, N(H), and/or the relative values of T_1, the interpulse time t_i (180°-90°), and the repetition time of the pulse sequence, t_r (180°-180°):

$$I = N(H)(1 - 2e^{-t_i/T_1}) + e^{-t_r/T_1}$$

In Figure 54 a series of images is shown made with the IR sequence for different t_i times. If T_1 is much longer than t_i the phase of the signal becomes negative. In other words, after the 90° read pulse in the first part of the relaxation curve the signal has a 180° phase difference. If the phase is incorporated in the image, the IR image would be 'inverted' in the first part of the relaxation curve; CSF would be white, and grey and white matter more grey.

In some machines this is indeed the case. However, it is also possible to measure the amplitude of the FID and ignore the phase. To illustrate this 'magnitude' or 'absolute value' reconstruction we have, in Figure 55, mirrored the first part of the relaxation curve: the signal

66

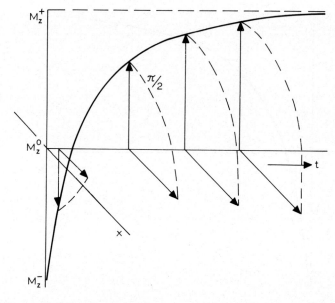

Figure 52. After a 90° ($\pi/2$) pulse the magnetization along the z-axis is nutated into the transverse plane and can be measured. In this representation the signal, originating from the negative part of the z-axis, is turned to the positive side of the x-axis, and therefore will give a positive signal, though the phases are in opposite directions. In this procedure, in which the phase is ignored, we speak of 'magnitude reconstruction'.

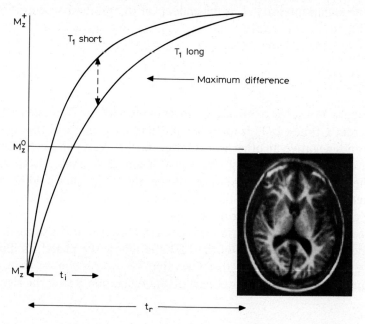

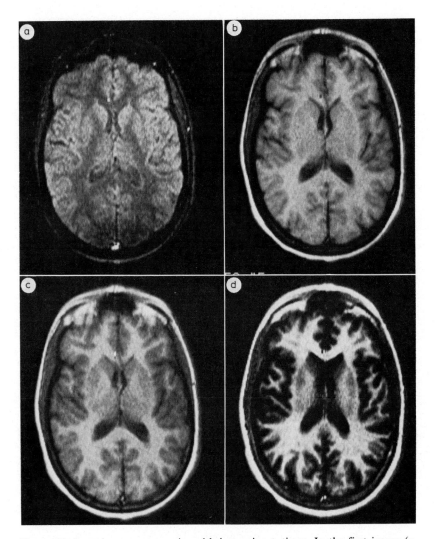

Figure 54. Inversion recovery series with increasing t_i times. In the first image (a, 100/1400) the magnetization is close to zero. With longer t_i times (b, 200; c, 300; d, 400 mseconds) the contrast between the tissue components increases.

Figure 53. Inversion recovery: return of the magnetization along the z-axis for two tissue components with different T_1 times. At a certain t_i the contrast is maximal. For the brain this is in the order of 400 mseconds.

intensity decreases in the first part of the trajectory and subsequently, after passage of the zero line (xy plane), increases. If we consider three tissue components with different T_1, then the points of transition between decreasing and increasing of the signal strength lie at different t_i times after the 180° pulse, t_1, t_2, t_3, respectively, for each of the tissues, i.e., white matter, grey matter and CSF.

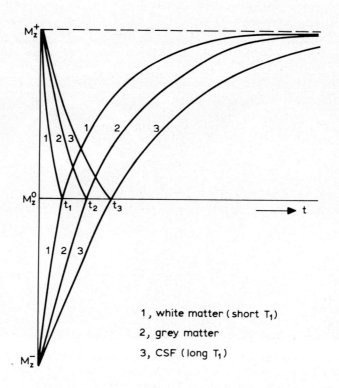

Figure 55. Inversion recovery relaxation curves for three tissue components: white matter, grey matter and CSF. White matter has the shortest T_1, CSF the longest. In this sequence a short T_1 gives a brighter signal. The first part of the relaxation curve is mirrored. It will be clear that in the mirrored image the CSF will have the brightest image until the relaxation curve crosses that of the white matter. It is also evident that in the area between t_1, t_2, t_3, many of these cross-overs occur, which can make assessment of the images awkward. If possible one should avoid this part of the curve.

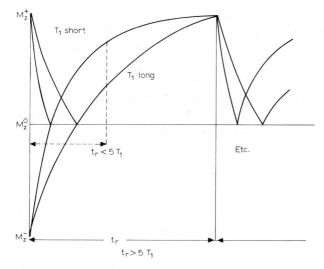

Figure 56. Inversion recovery: with $t_r > 5\,T_1$ all the magnetizations along the z-axis have been restored. The following 180° pulse is given at the same initial value as the first. If the t_r is much shorter than $5\,T_1$, illustrated on the left side of the figure, the initial values will not have been restored fully: tissue components with a relatively short T_1 have recovered more than tissues with a relatively long T_1.

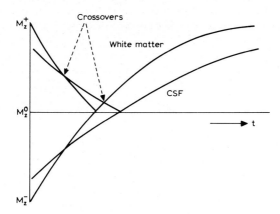

Figure 57. Representation of the exponential recovery of the magnetization along the z-axis of white matter (short T_1) and CSF (long T_1) in an IR sequence with $t_r \approx T_1$. Because the magnetization is not restored fully, the initial values have become unequal.

What has been said about t_r in the SR sequence also applies to the IR sequence. If one wants a new pulse sequence to start in an equilibrium situation, the t_r has to be at least 5 times the longest T_1 (Fig. 56). However, with regard to the acquisition time this is not practicable. To decrease the acquisition time one has to shorten the t_r. Of course, this has consequences for the imaging process (Fig. 56).

Let us assume that instead of $t_r = 5 \, T_1$ (this T_1 representing the tissue with the longest relaxation time) we chose $t_r = T_1$. The relaxa-

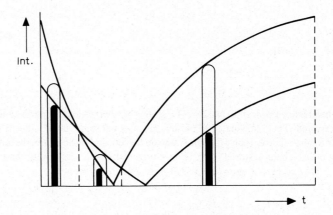

Figure 58. Relaxation curves at $t_r = T_1$ for two tissue components. In the first part the tissue with the shortest T_1 gives the brightest signal. Two contrast inversions occur during the relaxations of these two tissues (also see Fig. 59).

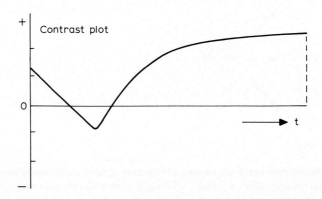

Figure 59. Contrast plot of the two tissue components of Figure 58, with $t_r = T_1$.

tion curves obtained in that case are drawn in Figure 57. Only two tissue components, white matter and CSF, are represented. Contrary to the sequence with $t_r \gg 5\,T_1$, here the tissue with the shortest T_1 has

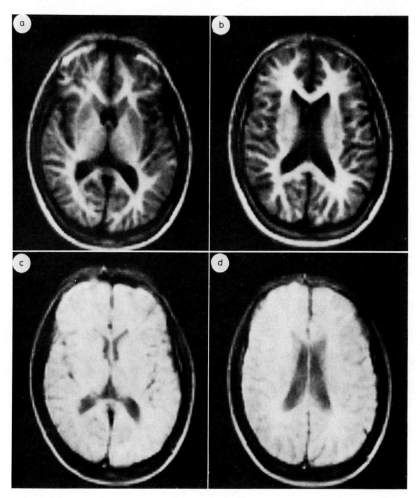

Figure 60. Difference in the nature of the images with IR and SE pulse sequences. a, b, Inversion recovery images at the level of the ventricles made with t_i = 400 mseconds and t_r = 1400 mseconds (IR 400/1400). Good separation of white and grey matter. c, d, Spin echo image at the same level with t_e = 50 mseconds and t_r = 2000 mseconds (SE 50/2000). In these T_2-dependent images the contrast difference between white and grey matter is small. However, the potential of this sequence to detect pathological tissue is greater than that of the IR sequence.

the brightest signal initially. When the contrast inverts, the tissue with the longest T_1 gives the brightest signal, and hereafter one more inversion occurs. Therefore, there are two 'cross-overs' in this sequence (Fig. 58).

For the imaging process the consequences are clear. The pulse sequence, t_i and t_r have to be known to allow correct interpretation of the images (see also in Fig. 60). Often the IR sequence is not the first choice, because experience has taught that the differences in T_2 relaxation times between healthy and pathological tissue are more prominent than differences in T_1. Therefore, the spin echo sequence is often used as a first choice, using multiple echo techniques.

IV SPIN ECHO

How spin echoes are generated has already been discussed in chapter 2. After a 90° pulse an FID can be registered. Because of the inhomogeneities of the field this decay is in general not a true measure of the spin-spin relaxation time, T_2. The spins dephase rapidly after the 90° pulse. They can be refocused by a 180° pulse. The signal increases again in strength. With regard to the original signal, however, it has decreased with a factor that is characterized by the 'real' relaxation time T_2 (Fig. 61). T_2 is, as is T_1, characteristic for a certain kind of tissue; it is only dependent on temperature, frequency and state of tissue; it is not a variable time. The pulse sequence can be schematically represented as:

spin echo

The spin echo has its maximum at a time $2 t_i$ ($= t_e$). The simple 90°-180° pulse sequence, however, can be extended by repeatedly applying 180° pulses; the echo intensity will then, obviously, decrease.

Experience has shown that, as previously mentioned, pathological

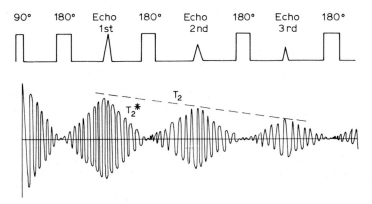

Figure 61. Multiple spin echoes; the signal intensity is measured at the peak of the echo. A number of measurements (at least two) define T_2. For the imaging process precise knowledge of T_2 is, of course, not necessary. The intensities of the first, second and third echoes are transformed directly into images.

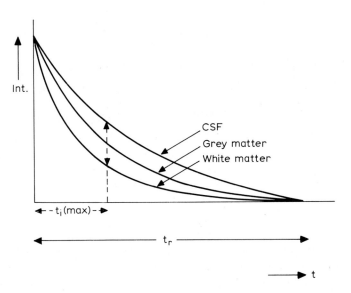

Figure 62. Decay curves of a series of spin echoes for white matter, grey matter and CSF. The CSF has the longest T_2. Measuring the relative values at a time t_i (max) leads to an image in which the CSF is bright, grey matter moderately grey and white matter dark grey.

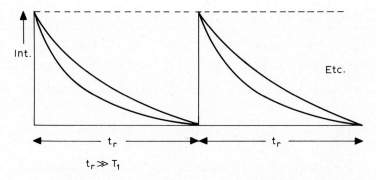

Figure 63. If t_r is chosen to be long enough ($t_r > 5\,T_1$) M_z has been restored fully for all tissue components. Each new pulse sequence starts at the same position. There are no 'cross-overs', the contrast relations (Fig. 64) remain the same.

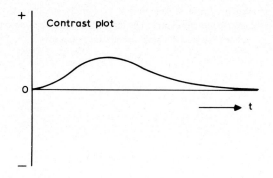

Figure 64. Contrast plot for SE sequence with $t_r \gg T_1$.

tissue can often be recognized best by later echos in the echo sequence. Therefore, it is important to have the facility to also image second and third order, etc., echo signals. The signal intensity is then low, but this has to be weighed against the greater specificity of the information. This pulse sequence also has the advantage of being the least time demanding. The relative signal strength of the various tissue components is dependent on both T_1 and T_2, in relation to the chosen t_r, the pulse repetition time. If t_r is long with regard to T_1 of the examined object, as is usual in the spin echo sequence, the images are mainly T_2-weighted. With a shorter t_r, however, the image becomes more

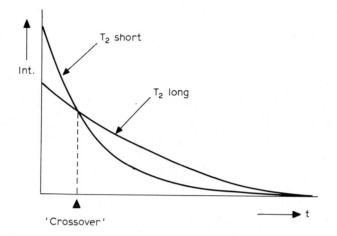

Figure 65. With a pulse sequence in which $t_r \approx T_1$ the magnetizations of the tissue components have not yet attained fully their equilibrium value. This leads to contrast inversion, 'cross-overs'. (As in the IR sequence, the contrast is zero at the cross-over point.)

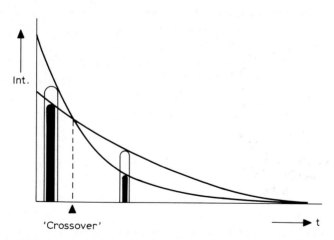

Figure 66. After cross-over, the tissue with the longer T_2 has the brighter signal.

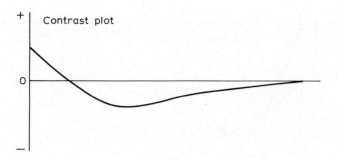

Figure 67. Contrast plot for two tissue components as in Figure 66.

dependent on T_1 because the magnetization along the z-axis has not been restored fully. From the equation

$$I = N(H) \, (1 - e^{-t_r/T_1}) \, e^{-t_e/T_2}$$

in which $N(H)$ is the proton density, t_r the pulse repetition time and t_e the echo time ($2 \times t_i$), these relations are clear. A shorter T_1, but especially a long T_2, gives a bright signal (high intensity) in the spin echo images. The image, as will be obvious from the previous discussion, can be manipulated by changing t_r and/or t_e. As for the SR and IR sequences the relaxation or decay curves for different tissue components can be graphically represented, as demonstrated for white matter, grey matter and CSF in Figure 62.

The graphs in Figure 62 show uncomplicated decay curves. It is simple to indicate the t_e at which the tissue T_2 differences are maximal. However, this graph represents a situation in which t_r is many times longer than T_1, for example, $\gg 5\, T_1$. Repetition of the pulse occurs with fully restored magnetization along the z-axis (Fig. 63).

In this case the M_z values of all tissue components with similar proton density are initially the same. The contrast plot shows a simple 'monophasic' curve (Fig. 64). Very often, for practical purposes t_r cannot be chosen to be larger than $5\, T_1$. The initial orientations of the tissue M_z values are then still influenced by their T_1 times. The initial M_z for tissue with short T_1 is greater than that of tissue with a longer T_1. The decay curves of the various tissues will now cross each other, leading to inversion of contrast, the so-called 'cross-overs' (Fig. 65). The contrast plot now has a 'biphasic' appearance, as is shown in Figures 66 and 67.

In Figure 68 a series of spin echo images with different t_r times is shown, together with the calculated decay curves for three tissue components. From the decay curves the contrast in the images can be predicted.

Experimentally, it is rather easy to estimate t_e and t_r from the cross-overs for healthy tissue components, as is true for the t_i times in the IR sequence. As mentioned previously, T_1 and T_2 values of pathological tissue are not known beforehand. The same is true for their cross-over points. At the cross-over points the contrast is zero (Fig. 70) and the tissue components cannot be distinguished. This explains the need for an image series with different t_e and/or t_r, so that the examiner can obtain an impression after a wide stretch of the decay curves (multiple echo series). It is evident that accurate knowledge of the formation of the SE images is mandatory in order to arrive at a correct diagnosis.

Therefore, a combination of a multiple-slice, multiple-echo technique is preferred by most researchers. In such a series, images with different t_e times in multiple slices can be reconstructed as desired. In Figure 71 the reconstructed echo images in one plane are illustrated. The 'cross-overs' are evident. The images after a t_e of 30 mseconds are T_2-dependent and the differences between shorter and longer T_2 times are imaged. In pathological tissue T_2 changes are more conspicuous than T_1 differences. For that reason the SE sequence, performed with multiple-slice, multiple-echo technique, is practised more and more as the method of choice for a first orientation (Fig. 72).

78

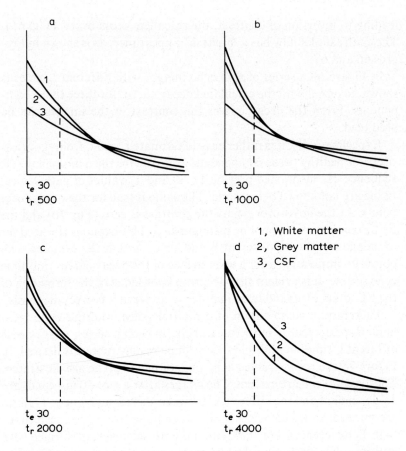

Figure 68. The decay curves correspond with the images on the right. With a constant t_e of 30 mseconds, the t_r is, respectively, 500, 1000, 2000 and 4000 mseconds. The highest signal intensity has the brightest colour in the image. The cross-over between CSF and

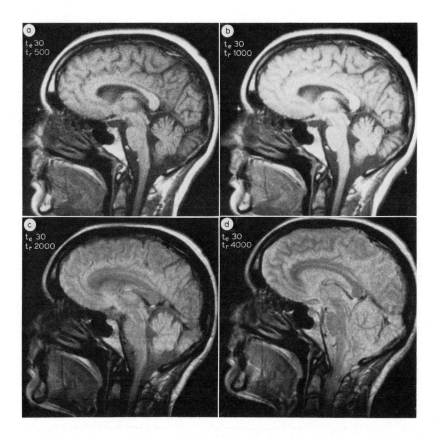

the other tissue components occurs at t_r times between 2000 and 4000 mseconds. In practice, more measurements can be made to obtain a favourable signal to noise ratio (Fig. 69).

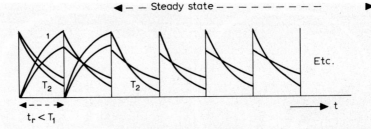

Figure 69. Repeated SE sequences with $t_r \approx T_1$. Registration starts after the system is in a steady state. The first measurements are ignored.

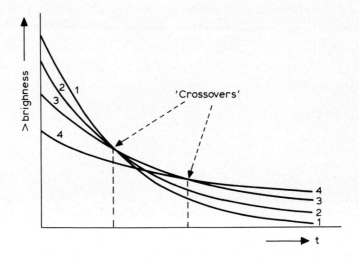

Figure 70. SE decay curves for white matter (1), grey matter (2), CSF (3) and pathological tissue with a longer T_2 (4). The cross-over point for the healthy tissue components is seen at the left side of the image. The cross-over point of the CSF and the pathological tissue lies far to the right. Note that in the area between these two indicated cross-over points the contrast differences are small, and difficult to identify. The pathological tissue will appear brighter than the adjacent tissue only with a long t_e.

Figure 71. Multiple echo scans at the same level in the axial plane: $t_r = 2000$ mseconds. The cross-over point is now seen between $t_e = 60$ and $t_e = 90$ mseconds. With $t_e = 240$ mseconds, only tissue with a very long T_2 is still visible.

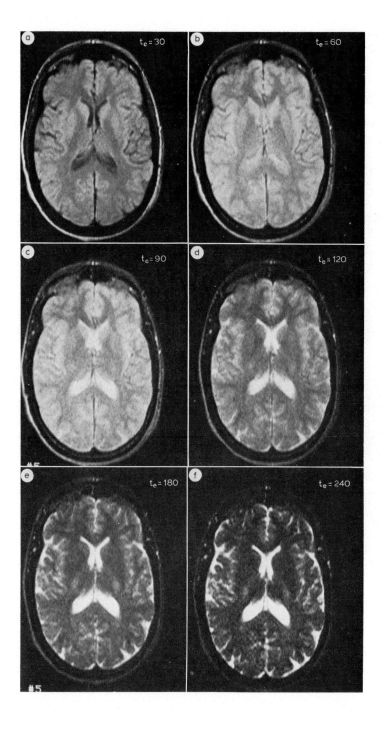

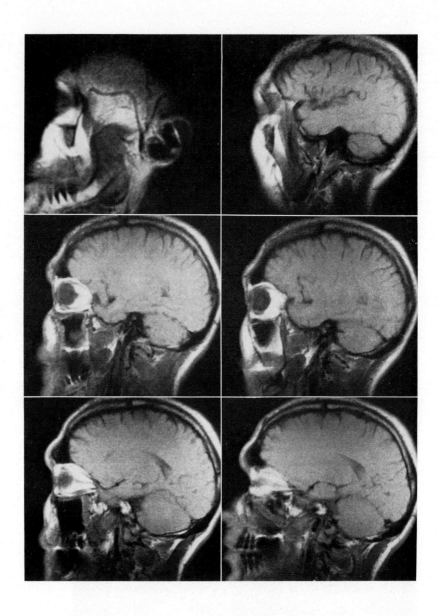

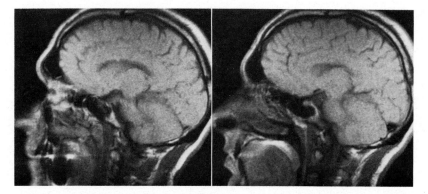

Figure 72. Multislice (multiecho) technique: 15 consecutive sagittal slices are made (in about 15 minutes), eight of which are shown in the figures, representing half of the head.

The localization of NMR signals in space

4

I   INTRODUCTION

In the previous chapter it was explained how the NMR imaging process can be manipulated by the choice of pulse sequences, and interpulse and repetition times. Obviously, it is necessary to localise the signals in space in order to make imaging possible.

In this chapter we deal with that aspect of imaging. A number of methods have been developed for the localisation of NMR signals three-dimensionally, thus allowing construction of images. Four such methods are discussed: 1, the sensitive point method; 2, the line techniques; 3, the imaging of a plane; 4, the imaging of a volume.

II   THE SENSITIVE POINT METHOD

In this method the static magnetic field is so arranged that only protons in a small volume, e.g., $3 \times 3 \times 3$ mm^3, satisfy conditions of resonance (Fig. 73).

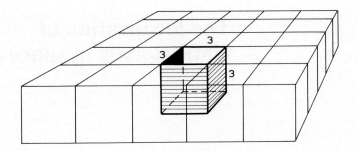

Figure 73. In the sensitive point method a magnetic field gradient is applied, so shaped that only protons in a small volume (voxel) are brought into resonance. To image other voxels, it is necessary to shift the object or the sensitive point from voxel to voxel. Of course, this method is very time consuming. In modern NMR imaging it is no longer used. However, it can still be used for topical NMR studies.

The point of sensitivity can be chosen by applying three static gradient fields in mutually perpendicular directions. These gradients are chosen in such a way that the resonance condition, $\omega = \gamma H_0$, only applies to a small volume. Protons outside this volume experience a magnetic field, not fulfilling the resonance condition. Therefore, they are not in resonance and do not give an NMR signal.

In terms of magnetization of protons in the rotating frame we can state that only in the sensitive point is the effective field identical to the RF field, H_1. For the partial magnetizations outside the sensitive point the effective field differs strongly from H_1 and the precession of the partial magnetizations does not occur around H_1, but around the effective field that they are subjected to. By an applied 90° pulse the partial magnetization vector of the voxels outside the sensitive point are deviated only weakly from the equilibrium direction; only the magnetization vector of the sensitive point turns 90° towards the transverse plane, and induces a free precession signal in the receiver coil.

To obtain images with this method the object has to be moved through this sensitive point, or vice versa. The method is then known as the 'sequential point' method. Of course, it is very time consuming, and cannot be used in clinical proton imaging. However, for spectroscopy (also in vivo) this method is still of value.

In the 'line' techniques a whole line from an object is imaged at the same time. For this method it is necessary to apply two gradient fields in mutually perpendicular directions, e.g., along the z-axis and the y-axis. Because of the gradient along the z-axis the magnetic field along this axis gradually increases, and therefore, according to the theorem of Larmor, also the resonance frequency of the nuclei. By now applying a 90° RF pulse with a well-defined frequency only one layer of nuclei reacts; this layer lies perpendicular to the direction of the gradient, the z-axis (Figs. 74 and 75).

The excited layer can now be considered isolated from the rest of the object and the problem is reduced to a two-dimensional problem. What has been done so far can be compared to the collimation of the X-ray beam in CT scanning. In CT scanning measurements are made under different angles, and by way of 'back projection' the image is

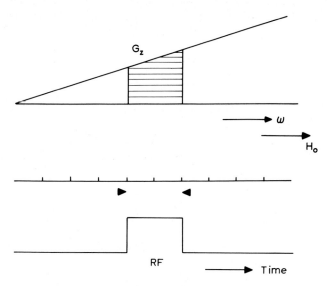

Figure 74. The gradient G_z is placed along the z-axis. After a 90° RF pulse only those protons which satisfy the Larmor resonance condition ($\omega = \gamma H_o$) resonate. In a field of 1 Tesla the resonance frequency of protons is 42.6 MHz. With an RF pulse of, for instance, 10^{-4} second, many oscillations of the RF field will still have taken place. Therefore, the RF frequency is well defined. If the pulse only contained one oscillation of the RF field then the frequency would be ill defined. With the pulse duration in use in NMR imaging this is not the case.

88

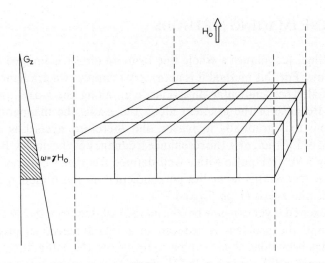

Figure 75. Application of a magnetic field gradient along the z-axis, and of an RF pulse with a well-defined frequency, defines a layer of protons that will resonate. The layers adjacent to this selected layer experience a different field, and therefore do not respond to the 90° RF pulse.

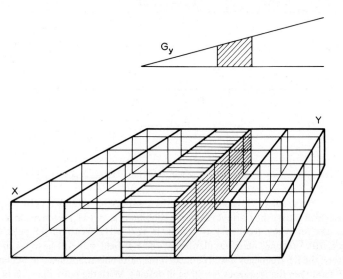

Figure 76. Selection of a line from a layer.

reconstructed. In NMR imaging this method can be mimicked by
shifting the gradient fields so that views from different angles are also
obtained (Fig. 78). However, in NMR imaging there are many ways
of solving localisation problems. For instance, we can, after having
selected a layer from the object (Fig. 75), apply a second gradient,
perpendicular to the first, e.g., along the y-axis. A 180° RF pulse is
now applied. Only those protons that satisfy the resonance condition
will respond. We obtain a spin echo signal only from those protons that
have reacted to the 90° RF pulse and subsequently to the 180° RF
pulse (Fig. 76). We have now defined a line in the object. To split up
this line into voxels (Fig. 77), a third gradient, along the x-axis, is
applied. Hereafter, it is possible to determine from the frequency spectra the position of the imaging points along that line. Along the line
there have to be as many echo registrations as there are imaging
points, imaged sequentially during the time the x gradient is applied.
The line can now be moved through the layer that has to be imaged by
shifting the gradients.

This method is obviously more efficient than the sensitive point
method, because it is not necessary to move the object or the sensitive
point to obtain an image of a layer.

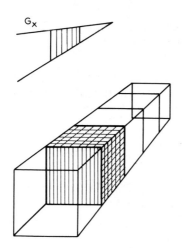

Figure 77. Selection of a voxel from a line.

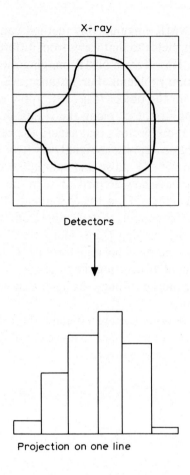

Figure 78. Projection on one line, as used in CT scanning. Similar projections on one line can be obtained in NMR imaging in a different way.

IV PLANE IMAGES BY BACK PROJECTION

In CT scanning the relative absorptions of the volume elements of the chosen slice are projected on one line (Fig. 78). By moving the X-ray tube and detectors around the object projections from different directions are obtained.

In CT scanning the image is now reconstructed from 'n' projections (Figs. 79 and 80). This is done by the 'back projection' method, or by

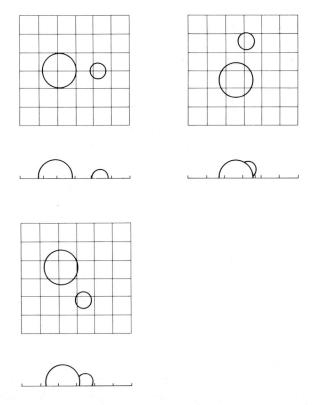

Figure 79. Projection on one line after turning the X-ray tube and detector system in CT scanning. From 'n' of these projections the image is reconstructed by filtered back projection. In this figure the object is turned instead of the X-ray detector system, as in the first CT scan experiments of Godfrey Hounsfield.

'filtered back projection'. In the latter case the object borders are accentuated in order to obtain a true reconstruction.

In NMR imaging the parameters are different from those in CT scanning: signal intensity, the phase of the induced signal and its frequency which is in accordance with the Larmor equation. The measured intensity is now distributed over a frequency spectrum. To achieve this it is necessary to apply a gradient in the direction in which one wants to determine the frequency distribution (Fig. 81). This frequency distribution is obtained after submitting the NMR signal to a Fourier transformation (Fig. 82).

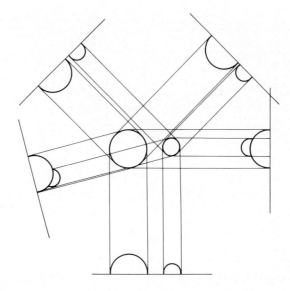

Figure 80. Reconstruction from the image shown in Figure 79 by back projection. In practice, during CT scanning 'filtered back projection' is used, with more accurate reproduction of the object.

In principle we now deal with the same situation as in the imaging process in CT scanning. However, to obtain images from different directions it is not necessary to rotate the system or the object. The projections can be obtained by step by step changing of the magnitudes of the gradient fields. With this method good images can be obtained, though the method is relatively slow, and is considered obsolete in NMR imaging. So far, one piece of information present in the NMR signal has not been discussed, the phase of the Larmor precession. This part of the NMR signal information can also be used to obtain spatial information. In this way two- and three-dimensional Fourier transformations are possible, leading directly to imaging.

Figure 81 (left). If no gradient is applied in the direction of the H_o field, no image of the spatial distribution is obtained. The different image lines cannot be separated.

Figure 82 (right). After the application of a gradient (G) the Fourier transformation of the FID gives spatial information. The Larmor frequency of the object on the right side is higher than that on the left side. In the receiving coil both precessions are detected; the summated signal shows the illustrated characteristic oscillation (see also Appendix 6).

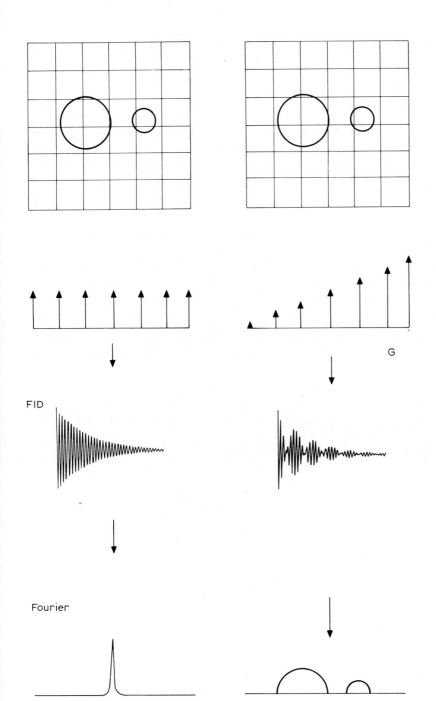

G

FID

Fourier

In two-dimensional Fourier analysis use is made of the phase of the precession of the magnetization. The first step is again selective irradiation of a slice of the object, so that one layer comes into resonance. All the partial magnetizations in the layer have, immediately after the pulse, the same phase. This is shown for a one line image in Figure 83. A field gradient is now applied during a certain period along one axis of the layer. Due to this 'phase-encoding' gradient differences in phase develop which are characteristic of the position in the object (Fig. 84).

Phase encoding has to be repeated as often as the number of voxels one wishes to image. In principle, it is possible to examine several slices at the same time, often with a small gap in between the slices for better separation of the NMR signals. Or consecutive slices are obtained by first scanning the odd slices and then the even ones. With such a multi-slice technique considerable time saving in acquisition is possible. The commercial systems now available offer up to 15 slices imaged simultaneously. The acquisition time of this multi-slice procedure is about 8–15 minutes, depending on the number of sequences.

Of course, it is necessary to apply a third gradient after the selection of a slice and a line. This third gradient finds the protons in a phase encoded by the second gradient. These phases are stored in the memory of the computer. Under influence of the third gradient the precessions accelerate or decelerate. This precession is in accordance with

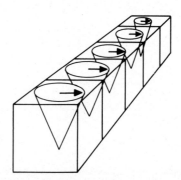

Figure 83. Immediately after the initial pulse the protons of the voxels in the layer are in phase, as shown here for one line in the irradiated layer.

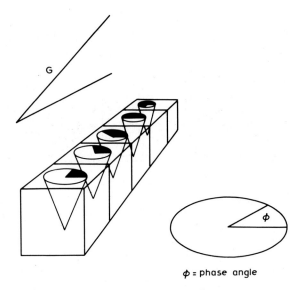

ϕ = phase angle

Figure 84. By applying a field gradient the precession frequency of the protons increases with the local magnetic field. The phase angle increases by an amount that is typical for the position of the voxels along the gradient axis. This means that the time during which the gradient is applied has to be determined precisely: the precession frequency is known, and therefore the phase angle per volume element. For obvious reasons, this type of gradient is called the 'phase-encoding' gradient.

the local field in the second gradient. The phase angle now obtained is the summation of the phase angles of the last two gradients (Fig. 85). This sequence is schematically represented in Figure 86.

To obtain data from all the imaging points it is necessary to step through as many phase-encoding gradient settings as there are image points along the y-axis. After each step an FID is collected. This FID is Fourier transformed and stored in the computer in as many increments as there are imaging points along the x-axis. The values of the corresponding data points along the x-axis for each gradient step also have a frequency pattern that now again is submitted to a second Fourier transformation, resulting in the image.

The possibility of direct imaging via Fourier transformation has been of great importance in the development of the NMR imaging system. This technique is now applied in multi-slice techniques for different pulse sequences. In Figure 86 a schematic representation is

96

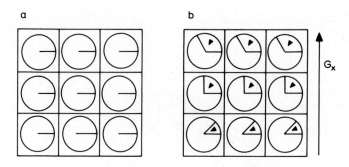

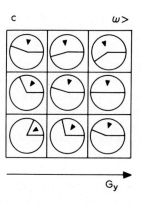

Figure 85. Two-dimensional Fourier analysis. a, After the initial pulse the phases of the proton magnetizations are equal. A slice is selected by G_z. b, Under influence of the gradient G_x, the protons localised in the direction of the gradient precess faster. After a certain time, t_x, position-dependent differences in phase angle have developed between the partial magnetizations. Perpendicular to the x-axis, however, the phases are identical. c, If a gradient along the y-axis is applied, the precession frequency of the magnetization along the y-axis is also dependent on this gradient. All places in the diagram are now characterized by phase and frequency.

given of the method just described. This method can be extended to include three dimensions. Instead of phase accumulations in two directions, the phases of three directions are accumulated.

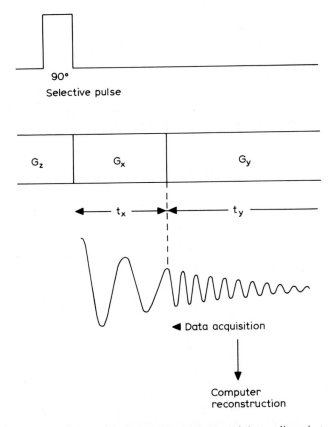

Figure 86. Schematic representation of the application of the gradients in two-dimensional Fourier analysis.

VI   THREE-DIMENSIONAL FOURIER ANALYSIS

In three-dimensional Fourier analysis a phase-encoding gradient is also applied in a second plane. The whole irradiated volume is then projected on one line, with encoding of the phases with respect to the other two axes. Of course, many more FIDs have to be collected to obtain the necessary information of each imaging point. The SR sequence of such a procedure is schematically represented in Figure 87.

If an SE sequence is used, the 90° RF pulse is followed by a 180° RF pulse and then the gradients are successively applied. Instead of vary-

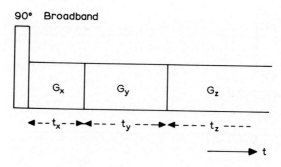

Figure 87. SE sequence for three-dimensional Fourier analysis.

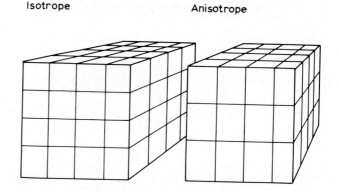

Figure 88. With three-dimensional Fourier analysis the same resolution can be obtained in all directions (isotrope). The acquisition time can be shortened by lessening the spatial resolution in one dimension (anisotrope).

ing the time of the gradients with small increments, the magnitude of the gradient can be varied while the duration is kept constant by a method called 'spin warping'. As already mentioned, to obtain the data of the image points of a whole volume many FIDs have to be collected. However, this results in a resolution which is the same in all planes; the resolution is isotropic. In cases in which one is only interested in the information in one direction the acquisition time can be shortened by accepting less accurate special information in one direction; the resolution is anisotropic (see Fig. 88). The three-dimensional Fourier analysis has as an advantage an optimal S/N because of the excitation of the whole volume, but the cost is a longer acquisition time.

NMRI equipment

5

I GENERAL REMARKS

The NMRI system is composed of a number of elements, each of which has a strong influence on the quality of the imaging process. The principal components are:

1. The magnet system; there are three types of magnet in use: permanent, electro-magnetic, and superconducting.

2. Shim coils, meant to improve the homogeneity of the static magnetic field.

3. Gradient coils, installed in three mutually perpendicular directions necessary to localize the NMR signal.

4. Coils for RF transmission and reception.

5. The system for data manipulation, amplifier, AD converter, computer, memory system, magnetic tape unit, matrix camera, display unit, etc.

These different components are shown in the architectural plans for an NMR site in an outpatient clinic of our hospital (Fig. 89). The reciprocal relations between the system components are shown in Figure 90. High-quality standards for each of the system components are mandatory. Development in the field of each of these subsystems can greatly influence image quality and patient handling.

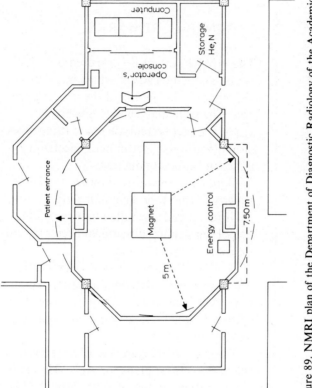

Figure 89. NMRI plan of the Department of Diagnostic Radiology of the Academic Hospital of the Free University, Amsterdam. The first zone of the magnetic field (30 Gauss) is contained within the magnet room.

He, N$_2$

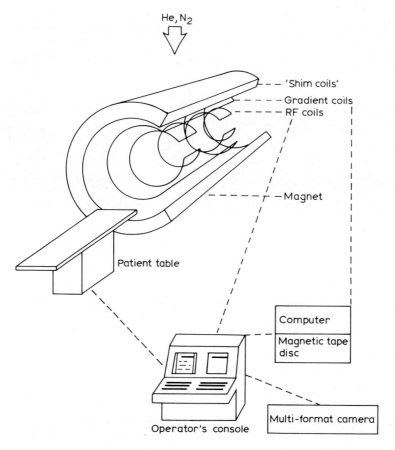

Figure 90. Schematic representation of the principal system components of an NMR imaging system.

II TYPE OF MAGNET

Three types of magnet are in clinical use:
Permanent magnets: these magnets are composed of 'permanent' magnetic material. The strength of the magnetic field depends on the nature and quantity of the magnetic material. For higher field strengths, weight is a real problem. An advantage is that permanent magnets need less shielding towards the environment because their fringe fields are weak. A second advantage is the absence of operating

102

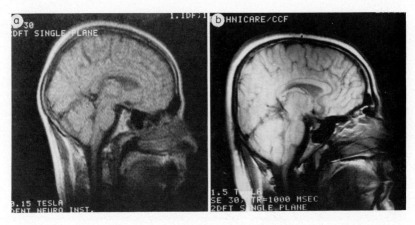

Figure 91. a, b, Comparison of two sagittal images made with a 0.15 Tesla resistive magnet (a) and a 1.5 Tesla cryomagnet (b). With the same acquisition time a much better S/N is obtained at 1.5 Tesla.

cost; the system does not need an external energy supply or cooling system to maintain the magnetic field. However, the homogeneity of the magnetic field is as a rule less than that obtained by superconducting magnets.

Electro-magnets: the magnetic field in an electro-magnet is produced by a current led through a number of windings. To obtain a fair homogeneity four coils are normally used, two large central ones and two smaller peripheral ones. The temperature of the windings is regulated by water cooling. The field strength usually lies between 0.15 and 0.35 Tesla; sufficient for proton imaging. With comparable acquisition time the S/N is far smaller than when stronger magnetic fields are used (Fig. 91). With adequate electronic equipment, however, images of reasonable quality can be obtained.

Cryogenic magnets: some metals and alloys become superconducting at temperatures close to absolute zero (0 Kelvin). The resistance in the magnetic windings is then zero and the current continues to flow without an external energy supply. Whole-body cryogenic magnets with homogeneous fields of 1.5–2 Tesla are commercially available at present.

The low temperature of the coils is maintained with liquid helium (boiling point 4.2 K), which is kept in a dewar. A buffer of liquid nitrogen (boiling point, 77.4 K) provides further insulation (Fig. 92).

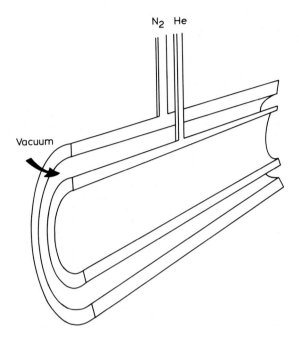

N₂ He

Vacuum

Figure 92. Schematic representation of the cooling components of a cryostatic magnet.
In modern magnets nitrogen cooling is not necessary because of better insulation.

In modern cryomagnets the insulation is so far improved that the
nitrogen buffer is no longer necessary. The 'boil-off' of helium is
reduced to about 1 litre per day. The cost of liquid helium, and, to a
lesser extent, of liquid nitrogen is high. Compared with the electro-
magnetic system, however, one saves on the energy costs. Helium and
nitrogen have to be topped up from time to time; however, the amount
necessary is now within reasonable limits.

A cryomagnetic system can 'quench'; i.e., because of local heating
the helium suddenly boils off and the magnetic field rapidly falls off.
The risk for the patient of this rapid change in magnetic field is considered to be small; the magnet has enough self induction to make the
change gradual; electronic circuits can also be installed to minimize
this small risk even further. The rapid movement of the head in and
outside the magnetic field, imitating quench, leads to the phenomenon
of magnetic phosphenes (light flashes) but this is inconsequential,
from a medical point of view. Higher magnetic fields subtend larger

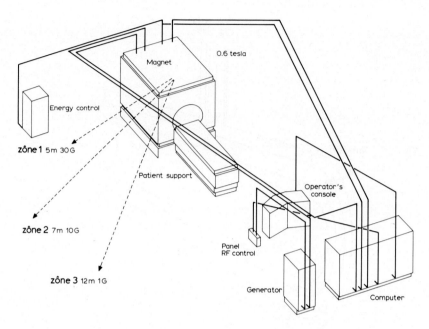

Figure 93. A 0.6 Tesla magnet and the magnetic zones that have to be taken into account.

Zones for a 0.6 Tesla cryomagnet (1 Tesla = 10,000 Gauss, 0.6 Tesla = 6,000 Gauss)*.

Zone 1: 5 meters≈30 Gauss
This zone should be out of bounds for all large ferromagnetic objects such as iron, O_2 and NO_2 cylinders, and smaller objects such as scissors, knives, instruments, etc. Patients with pacemakers should not be allowed into this area. The field strength may influence electronic equipment, computers and measuring devices, and will distort images on TV monitors. Magnetic information on credit cards may be erased; magnetic tape eventually will be wiped clean and watches may be damaged.

Zone 2: 7 meters≈10 Gauss.
The influence on the environment is considerably less, but the area is still restricted for patients with pacemakers and for electronic equipment.

Zone 3: 12 meters≈1 Gauss.
Further decay of the stray magnetic field. However, some influence on electronic equipment is still possible.

---

* For comparison: the strength of the earth's magnetic field is about 0.5 Gauss.

stray fields which may influence electronic equipment, monitors and measuring devices. The zones of the stray fields for a 0.6 Tesla magnet system are shown in the diagram in Figure 93.

Conversely, the environment may affect the imaging system. Steel in the construction of the building, elevators, streetcars, cars, radiofrequency transmissions, etc., have potentially disturbing effects on the imaging system. The site planning should take all these factors into consideration to guarantee an optimally functioning system. With increasing magnetic field strengths the zones will be proportionally larger. If necessary, it is possible to shield the magnetic field with respect to these factors.

It is not yet clear which magnetic field strength is optimal for whole-body proton imaging. Probably the compromise between S/N, acquisition time, and possible heating of the body at higher fields, will result in an optimal field strength of about 0.6–0.7 Tesla. Higher field strengths demand higher radiofrequencies. The stronger field also lengthens the T_1 and T_2 of tissue. Recently, it has been shown that proton imaging at 2.0 Tesla leads to less optimal images because of the chemical shift of 4 ppm of protons in H_2O relative to protons in aliphatic chains (CH_2). It is possible to image these two components separately, an advantage in some disease entities. However, the acquisition time will be increased. Much development in this field is to be expected in the coming years.

III COILS

The NMR imaging system is equipped with three types of coils. Shim coils are necessary to compensate for inhomogeneities in the static magnetic field, due partly to the magnet and partly to magnetic influences of the environment. This compensating field remains constant, of course, during the imaging process.

The linear changes in the magnetic fields, necessary to localize the NMR signals three-dimensionally, are provided by gradient coils along the x-, y- and z-axes. These gradient coils are, together with the shim coils, installed in the bore of the magnet. For each of the gradient coils a separate arrangement is necessary, so that each gradient can be switched on and off at the right time. In a pulse sequence of 0.5 second the gradients have to be applied successively for periods of 10 mseconds or less. To tip the magnetization over 90° or 180° a radiofrequency transmitter is necessary. The RF frequency is, of course, tuned to the frequency of the system: 42.6 MHz at 1 Tesla, 21.3 MHz for 0.5 Tesla, 6.39 MHz for 0.15 Tesla, etc.

The resonant signal of the protons is collected by a receiver coil. Often the same coil is used for transmission and reception, even though the difference in signal strength between the two is in the order of $1:10^3$. Most of the coils used in the imaging equipment are of a relatively simple shape. The optimal length of the RF coil is a function of the wavelength of the signal at the field strengths used in NMRI, ($\lambda = 14.1$ m at 0.5 Tesla, 46.9 m at 0.15 Tesla). The geometry of the coils is of great importance to obtain an optimal signal to noise ratio. The 'filling' factor of the coil is another important aspect in the quality of the received signal. For this reason smaller coils are used for the head than for the body. Conditions for the body are less favourable. The filling is less homogeneous, and, because of the necessarily larger size of the coil with the same imaging matrix, there is a decrease in spatial resolution. These conditions make it necessary to use larger field gradients at higher magnetic field strengths. The higher RF frequencies lead to greater heat dissipation into the body. In practice this means that multi-slice techniques in the body can be hampered by induced currents and heating of the body. The longer T_2 at higher field strengths has a disadvantageous effect on acquisition time. The normal gain in S/N obtained at higher field strengths can thus be lost, and there seems to be, at the present state of art, an optimum of about 0.7 Tesla for NMR body imaging, combining a reasonable image quality and an acceptable throughput of patients (D.I. Hoult, 1984).

IV SURFACE COILS

The development of high-quality coils will certainly have a great influence on the quality of NMRI in the near future. A significant improvement in S/N is possible by the use of surface coils. These coils can be brought into close contact with the region of interest, with a considerable improvement of S/N. They can be used to give detailed images of the eye, the petrous bone, the spine, the heart, parts of the

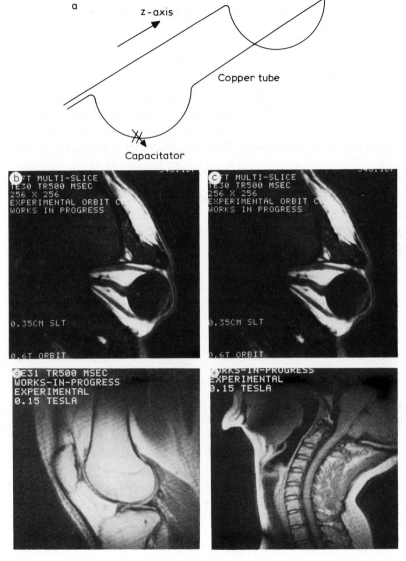

Figure 94. a, Possible shape of a surface coil. The length is in the direction of the z-axis (= axis of the magnet), so that as much as possible of the transverse magnetization can be detected. The coil has to be adapted to the system and tuned at the frequency of the system. b, c, Images of the contents of the orbit obtained with a surface coil. The improvement in detail is considerable. d, Sagittal image of the knee made with a surface coil on a resistive system (0.15 T). e, Sagittal image of the neck, made with a surface coil on a resistive system (0.15 T). The intervertebral discs and the myelum are shown well. Good detail is also obtained in the larynx and epiglottis region.

extremities, the breast, etc. Surface coils are always receiver coils, the transmitter coil of the system remains unchanged. It is possible to make surface coils of copper or silver wire, with a simple geometry and fitted with a capacitator to tune the coil to the resonant frequency of the system (Fig. 94a). Though the construction is relatively simple, there are some potential dangers in the use of surface coils, and therefore the installation and handling of such coils is better left to experts. Figures 94b and c demonstrate the improvement of quality that can be obtained with this type of coil. Surface coils will doubtless also play an important role in 'in vivo' spectroscopy in the coming years. However, this demands a good S/N as well as local magnetic field homogeneity of $\geq 1:10^6$. Penetration of the region of interest with surface coils is limited to an area not much deeper than the radius of the coil. However, this limitation of area can also be an advantage.

Contrast agents for NMR

6

I INTRODUCTION

Contrast media play an important role in conventional diagnostic radiology. They make it possible to differentiate between tissue components that otherwise would be indistinguishable. They are given intravascularly, orally or via enemas. The intravascular compounds contain iodine atoms in a complex molecule; in oral and pre-rectal applications barium is usually used as a contrast agent. To a more limited extent, 'negative' contrast media such as air or oxygen are used, e.g., in O_2 meatography during CT scan. The improvement in information is the result of the visualization of structures, organs, and blood vessels that were of about equal density (isodense) as the surrounding tissue before the administration of the contrast agent. Such 'contrast' examinations include the stomach, intestine, gallbladder, blood vessels, collecting system of the kidneys, etc. Contrast enhancement often causes visualization of pathological tissue with a specific affinity for contrast or which has a defective barrier, e.g., the blood-brain barrier. After contrast

110   administration the target object of the investigation will stand out from its surroundings because of a greater or smaller absorption of X-rays than in the surrounding tissues. The increase in X-ray absorption is the result of the different electron density of the contrast medium.

Compared with contrast agents used in diagnostic radiology, NMR contrast agents show both similarities and differences. Just as in conventional diagnostic radiology, the role of NMR in the near future will be influenced greatly by the ability of contrast media to improve the range and efficiency of NMR studies and to improve tissue characterization (e.g., oedema versus tumour). In the first place, NMR contrast agents are meant to distinguish tissue components with identical NMR characteristics, and in the second place to shorten the relaxation times.

Just as in X-ray pyelography or enhanced CT studies of the kidney, renal excretion can be assessed by intravenous injection of paramagnetic contrast material in NMRI. These paramagnetic substances locally affect the relaxation of the protons, and hence the contrast in the image, producing a visible result. An important difference between X-ray contrast media and NMR contrast agents is the direct involvement in the imaging process of the X-ray contrast medium and the indirect method of enhancement by NMR contrast agents. The extent to which the signal strength is affected by an X-ray contrast medium is a linear function of the concentration. The complicated indirect

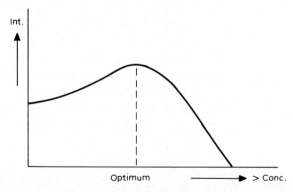

Figure 95. The concentration of a paramagnetic substance plotted against the intensity of the effect shows an optimum concentration with maximum effect on the NMR signal.

influence on the image of an NMR contrast agent leads to an optimum concentration (Fig. 95) at which the enhancing effect is best seen. The different types of contrast agents that can be used in NMR have the common characteristic that they locally enhance the fluctuating fields, so that the relaxation times T_1 and T_2 become shorter. A shorter T_1 may lead to a stronger signal; a shorter T_2, however, leads to a lower intensity signal. These two contradictory influences are among the factors which cause the non-linearity of concentration and signal strength in the use of NMR contrast agents.

We shall mention only briefly the possibility of influencing the NMR image by using hydration and dehydration to change proton density. The practical use of these procedures is limited.

II   PARAMAGNETIC IONS

A paramagnetic substance consists of molecules that possess one or more unpaired electrons. Like ferromagnetic materials, paramagnetic substances are attracted by a magnetic field, but to a lesser extent. Not all materials are paramagnetic. On the other hand, all molecules and atoms are diamagnetic; by virtue of its magnitude, paramagnetism can mask diamagnetism.

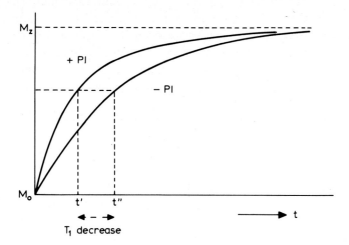

Figure 96. Relaxation curves with and without the presence of paramagnetic ions (PI). In this case, the shorter T_1 in the presence of paramagnetic ions is clear.

A diamagnetic substance is repelled by a magnetic field because the field induces circular currents that can be regarded as magnetic dipoles opposing the field. These dipoles are proportional to the field. In standard imaging fields they are, in magnitude, comparable to the magnetic dipole moments of magnetic nuclei. The magnetic moments of unpaired electrons are roughly 10^3 larger than those of protons.

In diamagnetic molecules all electrons are paired; in this case there are no dipole fields originating from unpaired electrons. In the vicinity of paramagnetic molecules a weak dipole field is present, varying from time to time and from place to place: therefore, the dipole field fluctuates. Such a field can be very effective in shortening the relaxation times T_1 and T_2 of nearby protons (Fig. 96). This is understandable when one realises that the time-dependent dipole field can contain frequencies close to the Larmor frequency of the protons in the tissue. It is clear that with a shorter T_1 the signal intensity stabilises more quickly than with a longer T_1. A shorter T_2 accelerates the decay of the echo amplitude. From the signal intensity equation during the SE sequence:

$$I = N(^1H)\,(1 - e^{-t_r/T_1})\,e^{-t_r/T_2}$$

Depending on the repetition rate, one can therefore infer that I increases with shorter T_1, while a shorter T_2 tends to weaken the signal intensity (shorter $T_1 \rightarrow\, >$signal intensity; shorter $T_2 \rightarrow\, <$signal intensity). It is obvious that extensive research has been done on the possibilities of paramagnetic substances in nuclear magnetic resonance imaging, in vitro and also in vivo, including in human beings. Substances which potentially could be used (after Brasch, 1983) are:

1. Molecules with unpaired electrons: nitric oxide (NO); nitrogen dioxide (NO_2); molecular oxygen (O_2).

2. Ions with unpaired electrons: these are ions from the 'transition series'; in the first series the so-called 3-d orbit is completed, in the Lanthanides series the 4-f orbit, etc. Ions from the first series are: Mn^{2+}, Mn^{3+} (manganese); Fe^{2+}, Fe^{3+} (iron); Ni^{2+} (nickel); Cr^{2+} (chromium); Cu^{2+} (copper).
The Lanthanide series: in principle all Lanthanides are fit for application, with the exception of lanthane and lutetium. Research with

NMR imaging is mainly done with: Gd^{3+} (gadolinium) and Eu^{3+}
(europium).
The Actinide series: Pa^{4+} (palladium).

3. Stable free radicals: (strictly these compounds belong to category 1). In NMR imaging use is often made of 'nitroxide stable free radicals' (NSFR). The stable nitroxide radical can be built into other molecules. Examples are: pyrrolidine NSFR and piperidine NSFR. For most of the substances the toxicity is such that they cannot be used clinically without further elaboration.

III BIOLOGICAL TOLERANCE

The problem with all potential NMR contrast agents is their toxicity when used in human beings. However, recently this problem seems to have been overcome with respect to a number of contrast agents. Chelates of iron, and especially of gadolinium, with ethylene diamine tetraacetic acid (EDTA) and diethylamine triamine pentaacetic acid (DTPA) has lowered toxicity considerably. Gadolinium DTPA has been linked to two meglumine molecules with many hydrophyl groups, resulting in an NMR contrast agent that has already been used successfully (Fig. 97). Of course, this will have a great impact on the further clinical development of NMR imaging.

After successful completion of phase 1 and 2 experiments with gadolinium-chelate-dimeglumine, the third phase with clinical trials on volunteers and patients also appears to be successful. The effect on

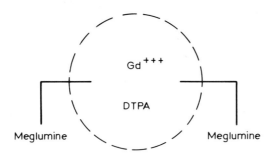

Figure 97. Gadolinium-chelate-dimeglumine (developed by Schering, F.R.G.), a contrast agent for NMRI that can be used intravenously.

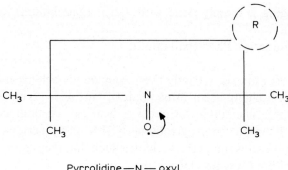

Pyrrolidine—N—oxyl

Figure 98. The structural formula of a stable free radical of the nitroxide type; the unpaired electron on the O atom is protected from reactions in the pyrrolidine complex. In the R position, biologically interesting groups càn be substituted.

NMR signals is evident from these experiments. The future will show if it is possible, using these contrast agents, to differentiate tissue components more effectively than hitherto, for example, cerebral tumours from surrounding oedema.

Several reports to this effect have been published recently. Another group of contrast agents with future possibilities is the group of nitrogen stable free radicals, as was already mentioned (Fig. 98). When a method can be found to use these compounds safely in humans, they could be valuable as spin-label compounds, as has been shown in animal experimentation. In this way it may become possible to produce tissue-specific contrast agents (monoclonal antibodies), which could lead to another minor revolution in NMR imaging.

The clinical applications of NMR tomography

7

I INTRODUCTION

In this chapter we will review the current status of NMR tomography as a diagnostic imaging technique. The following is clearly intended to be a 'freeze frame'. As was discussed extensively in the previous chapters, changes are to be expected in the entire field. At this moment the diagnostic significance of NMR imaging is most clearly evident in neuroradiology. The head and spinal column have proved to be ideally suited to the NMR technique. The diagnostic prospects of NMR for the heart and mediastinum are promising. Cardiac gating appears to be making an important contribution in the diagnostic assessment of the cardiovascular system. The utilization of respiratory gating has been hampered by the slower and more irregular nature of the respiratory cycle. The state of the art in NMR technology with regard to the imaging of diverse organs and systems will be discussed and, where possible, a brief sketch of anticipated developments will be presented.

NMR, skull and cranial contents

The advent of CT scanning has proved to be of revolutionary significance in the diagnosis of intracranial pathology. A few fundamental problems remain. Areas adjacent to the cranium, portions of the posterior fossa where beam-hardening and volume averaging artefacts occur are often inadequately depicted. NMR has here a number of advantages. Cortical bone, for example, due to its relatively low mobile hydrogen (proton) content, generates a weak signal, and as such induces no artefacts. Therefore, bone is visualized as black; the subcutaneous fat (relatively short T_1, relatively long T_2) generates a strong signal and is visualized as white. When Fourier analysis is used in NMR imaging, the susceptibility to motional artifacts is significantly less than that of CT scanning. The CT scan can generate coronal and sagittal sections using either direct CT techniques or CT reconstructions from multiple transverse sections. The reconstructed images, however, suffer from a lack of adequate spatial resolution. Further image degradation can occur due to patient movement between scans. Direct sagittal and coronal CT sections are limited by gantry and table construction, and often require repositioning of the patient. The detection of NMR is fundamentally three-dimensional. NMR signals can be obtained from the entire volume contained between transmitter and receiver coil and the gradients changed at wish. Direct sagittal and coronal sections with good spatial resolution can therefore be made without repositioning the patient (see Figs. 102 and 103). Even with small difference in H_2O in the tissues sizeable differences in T_1 or T_2 can exist and be utilized for optimal contrast. Therefore a sharper discrimination between two tissues, e.g., the grey and white matter, can be obtained (Fig. 99) than is possible in CT studies.

The superiority in discrimination is currently such that cryomagnetic NMR systems are capable of visualizing structures such as the substantia nigra and red nucleus. We here reiterate that it is sometimes necessary to sacrifice visualization of anatomic detail in order to achieve a clinically more relevant discrimination between diseased and healthy tissue.

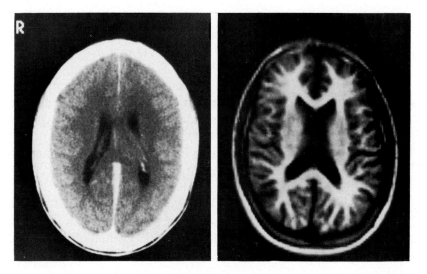

Figure 99. Comparing the CT scan and the NMR image (IR), the distinction in depicting grey-white differences is illustrated clearly between these two modalities.

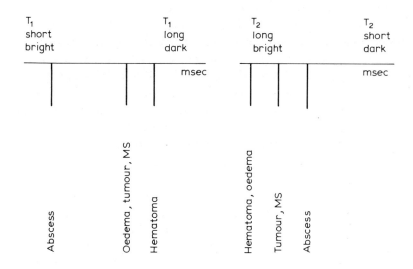

Figure 100. Pathological structures in vivo can be classified according to their T_1 and T_2, so that, eventually, characterization of the lesion can follow.

Figure 100 illustrates that T_1 and T_2 influences on the image at a certain pulse sequence can have such cancelling effects that contrast between tissues is lost. Therefore, it is almost always necessary to use more than one pulse sequence. When the T_1 and T_2 relaxation curves for two tissue components exhibit an identical course, discriminating between the two becomes impossible. It has already been established, for instance, that it is sometimes difficult to distinguish clearly between tumour and surrounding oedema. The immediate future will reveal whether NMR contrast media or tumour proton labeling can lead to a better discrimination capability in this respect. The effect will probably be comparable to contrast enhancement on the CT scan.

The ease with which sagittal sectioning can be obtained makes NMR scanning ideally suited for analyzing the soft tissues at the craniocervical junction. Therefore, the diagnostic evaluation of Chiari malformations, syringobulbia and syringomyelia is simplified considerably.

Specific applications

Intra-cerebral vascular conditions. The changes occurring after a cerebral infarction are evident much earlier on NMR images (as early as 90 minutes) than on CT images, where during the first 24 hours little change is discernible. Although little mention is made of it in the literature, it seems plausible that in transient ischaemic attacks (TIA) abnormalities may frequently be revealed by NMR scanning. CT findings are negative in 75–80% of these cases. How far this will be clinically relevant remains an open question, if a direct link with the prognosis is not established. The same consideration applies to complete strokes, and infarcts with neurological sequelae. The image series in Figure 101 illustrates the difficulty in discriminating between infarction, tumour and porencephalic cyst, using NMR. Images acquired using a spin echo technique with 50 mseconds t_e are not capable of depicting the difference between normal and abnormal structures. Only the IR images reveal the abnormality.

Perhaps a later echo ($>$ 60 mseconds) would have revealed the lesion. The example shows clearly the necessity of more than one pulse sequence.

Demonstrating intracranial haematomas is a simple matter using CT. Determining the prognosis on the basis of CT images, however,

has proved to be unsuccessful. In the diagnosis of cerebro-vascular
accidents, where the distinction has to be made between infarct and
hemorrhage, it does not seem likely that at its current stage of development NMR will supplant CT as the modality of choice. An 'explo-
ratory' CT examination in the batch-mode requires 10–15 minutes,
every slice takes about 4.5 seconds. A similar examination on the
NMR scan using two pulse sequences, IR and SE, or multiple echo
scan requires 30 minutes (15 minutes with the newer software).

The patient must remain immobile during this whole period. Even if
this requirement could be met, it is doubtful whether NMR could

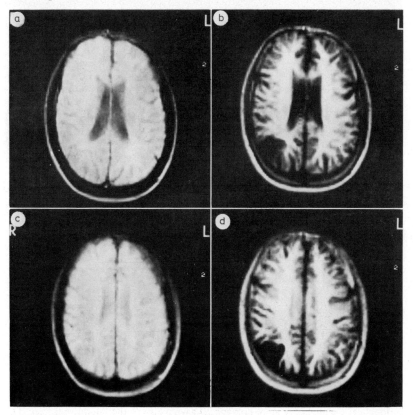

Figure 101. Comparison of SE and IR techniques in a postcontusional lesion (to be
differentiated from infarction and tumour). a, c, SE images (50/1500) at two levels. No
lesion becomes obvious. b, d, IR images (400/1400); the loss of tissue in the right pari-
eto-occipital region is now obvious. The images concur with the diagnosis of posttrau-
matic lesion.

improve upon the characteristic CT findings in, e.g., subarachnoidal bleeding. These are virtually diagnostic.

Isodense subdural haematomas. One of the problems with CT, though to a much lesser degree with current generation CT scanners, is the detection of isodense subdural haematomas. Although the issue

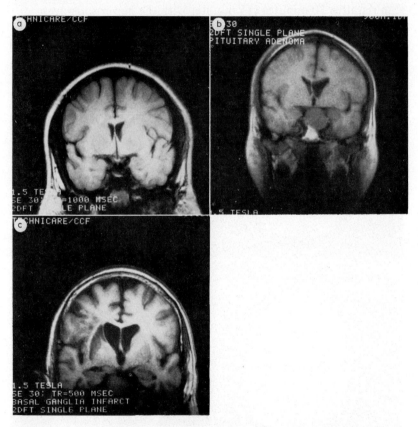

Figure 102. Selected coronal sections made with the 1.5 Tesla Technicare system, SE (t_e = 30, t_r = 1000 mseconds). Normal image, slight asymmetry of the lateral ventricles. b, Identical technique. A more pronounced asymmetry of the lateral ventricles. The optic chiasma and interpenduncular cisterns are filled with a mass originating in the vicinity of the pituitary gland. Compression of the optic chiasm; erosion of the sellar floor. c, SE (t_e = 30, t_r = 500 mseconds). Illustrates an old infarct located in the globus pallidus. The lateral ventricle has widened in the direction of the infarct. The cortical changes are also attributable to tissue loss.

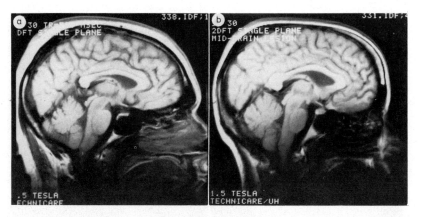

Figure 103. Among the most striking neurological images produced by NMR technique are the sagittal sections through the head that are obtained without the need to reposition the patient. We present two examples made with the 1.5 Tesla Technicare system. a, SE (t_e = 30, t_r = 500 mseconds): normal sagittal section. b, Identical technique: a lesion located in the mesencephalon with a low signal intensity and little mass-effect (infarct).

can usually be decided by observing a mass-effect or by administering intravenous contrast, isolated pitfalls leading to errors of interpretation are still possible. NMR imaging techniques are able to depict isodense subdural haematomas easily.

Tumours. It was noted in previous sections that it can sometimes be difficult to distinguish between tumour and oedema. In general, tumours are clearly visible, generating a high intensity signal when T_2-weighted sequences are used (Figs. 103 and 104). However, oedema also generates a similar signal. It has been demonstrated recently that intravenous injection of gadolinium DTPA helps to differentiate between tumour and oedema. Furthermore, the multiple echo/multiple slice sequences have proved to be useful in this respect. An exception to the rule that NMR has greater sensitivity for tumour detection than CT is formed by meningeomas. Sometimes these can be missed completely on the NMR study.

Another major limitation of NMR to date, in comparison to CT, has been its inability to visualize calcified structures directly. Calcifications can at best be inferred as a focus of partial signal drop-out. Certain tumours containing calcifications may not show them when scanned on NMR instead of a CT scanner. This is so in, for example,

122

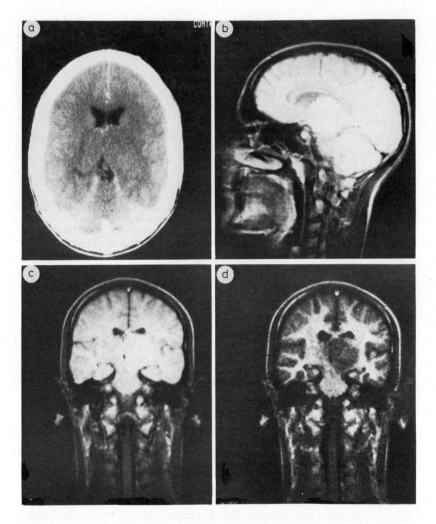

Figure 104. Analysis of a central lesion; comparison between CT scan and NMR scan. a, CT scan at the level of the thalamus discloses an isodense mass displacing the third ventricle to the right and indenting the pars media of the left lateral ventricle. The mass remains isodense after contrast injection. b, Spin echo NMR image (t_e = 50, t_r = 1500 mseconds) shows a sharp delineation of the lesion from its surroundings. The histological diagnosis was a low-grade oligodendroglioma. c, Coronal section (t_e = 100, t_r = 1500 mseconds). Spin echo depicts the lesion as a region of higher signal intensity than the surrounding tissues. T_2 value distinctly prolonged in the region of the lesion. d, The T_1-weighted IR images (t_i = 400, t_r = 1400 mseconds) depict the lesion as a region of low signal intensity, indicating a prolonged T_1. Prolonged T_1 and T_2 values are a common finding in pathological cerebral processes.

craniopharyngioma, necessitating an additional CT scan to establish the diagnosis. Tissue characterization using NMR is not developed fully enough to allow histologic diagnosis. The question remains open as to whether the implementation of paramagnetic contrast agents, in vivo NMR spectroscopy, or proton-labeled antibodies will make this feasible.

NMR has great potential in the diagnosis of pituitary tumours. The relation of the tumour to the basal cisterns, optic nerves and optic chiasm is visualized convincingly on NMR. The surveillance during pregnancy of the larger pituitary adenomas (which tend to grow) becomes possible, without subjecting the patient to X-rays or repositioning to obtain sagittal or coronal sections (Figs. 102–105). NMR images are not degraded by artefacts, unlike the CT scan images, and

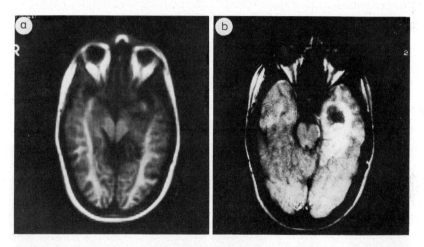

Figure 105. NMR analysis of a patient with temporal lobe epilepsy. These NMR images (using IR and SE techniques) were obtained from a 17-year-old girl suffering from incinate fits (olfactory hallucinations as the aura of a temporal lobe epileptic attack). a, The IR (400/1400) image shows a lesion generating a low signal intensity in the left unco-hippocampal region (T_1 prolongation). b, The SE (50/1500) image reveals a more extensive lesion in the same region with a predominantly higher signal intensity. The area of low intensity in this region probably represents a cyst within the lesion. Oedema, which generates a high signal intensity, could also account for this configuration. However, a mass-effect is missing, and the gyri of the hippocampus remain intact. The histological findings established an inactive spongioblastoma (hamartoma), in marked contrast to the normal macroscopic aspect (except for a colour difference) of the hippocampus encountered during operation. This type of lesion has a generally favourable prognosis.

display to better advantage the distinction between intra- and extra-axial tumours of the posterior fossa. In general, para-pontine and cerebello-pontine angle tumours can be distinguished clearly from intra-pontine, mesencephalic, fourth ventricle, vermis and cerebral hemisphere tumours. It goes without saying that 'indirect' tumour indicators, such as hydrocephalus, mass-effects and herniations, are depicted well on NMR images.

Infections. Initial publications have indicated that NMR imaging techniques may be useful in the diagnostic evaluation of infections. Here, too, it remains to be seen whether the information obtained is specific enough to allow one to go beyond the mere discernment of nondescript lesions causing a mass-effect. Viral infections such as herpes encephalitis appear to manifest themselves through a longer T_1 and T_2. If the diagram in Figure 100 is correct then abscess formation having a shorter T_1 and a longer T_2 can be discriminated from tumour tissue. The effect of paramagnetic contrast agents on NMR imaging of infectious processes is unknown at this moment.

White matter disease. NMRI is very promising in the diagnosis of white matter disease, given optimal resolution of white-grey matter

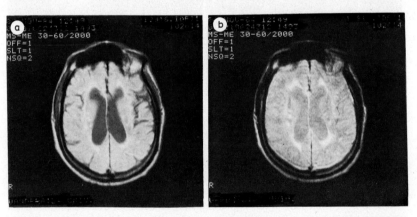

Figure 106. a, b, Spin echo images of a patient with white matter disease; 30/2000 and 60/2000. On the later SE scan the lesions around the ventricular system are seen better. It has become obvious that white matter affections are often seen in elderly people, though it is too early to assume that the disease named after Binswanger occurs even more often than was suspected from CT studies. Similar lesions can be seen in multiple sclerosis.

difference. The white matter, rich in triglycerides, usually has a strong signal. This high-intensity signal changes in cases in which the myelin is broken down, as in multiple sclerosis and the leuko-encephalitides. Usually both T_1 and T_2 lengthen (Fig. 106). The change in T_2 especially, makes the lesion visible in delayed SE scans. In multiple sclerosis NMRI demonstrates lesions that are not seen on CT. Recently, MS lesions have been demonstrated in the mesencephalon and pons. Disturbances in myelinisation in premature infants can be followed up with NMR, perhaps giving a better understanding of the late consequences of such findings, which tend to 'normalize' early on the CT scan.

Malformations. It is evident that the anatomical NMR images in axial, coronal and sagittal planes simplify an exact diagnosis of con-

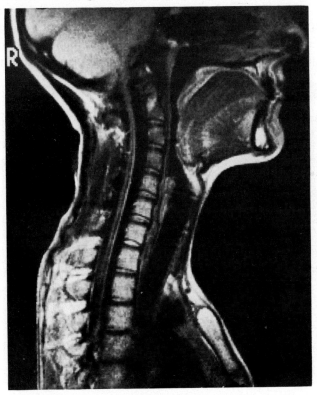

Figure 107. Sagittal section (50/1500) in the region of the cranio-cervico-thoracic spine. This patient has been operated upon for a Chiari 2 malformation with syringomyelia. The remnant of the syrinx can be seen clearly.

126   genital brain malformations. This is true for the whole gamut of cerebral malformations, as already proven, especially in the prosencephal-
ies, the lissencephalies, agenesis of the corpus callosum and vermis, the
Dandy Walker malformations, schizencephalies, porencephalies, etc.
Extensive experience exists with the Chiari 2 malformation and the
syringobulbia-syringomyelia complex. Sagittal NMR views demonstrate these lesions in a unique way (Fig. 107). Additionally, follow-up
of these patients is made much easier by NMR. However, one disadvantage is that bony anomalies are shown less well than on conventional X-ray tomography and CT scans.

Spinal canal and myelum. The NMR signals of cerebrospinal fluid
(CSF) and myelum are so different, given the right choice of pulse
sequence, that it is possible to obtain adequate images of the myelum
and the arachnoid spaces in the sagittal plane. According to the chosen
pulse sequence, the CSF can be depicted darker or lighter. It is important to check that the patient does not have a severe scoliosis. In such

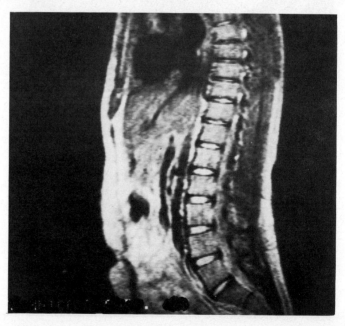

Figure 108. Sagittal images (60/2000) of the thoraco-lumbar area. The relatively long
T_2 gives the nucleus pulposus a bright signal, the cord is white and the CSF black, With
a longer t_e the CSF becomes white (relatively long T_2).

cases a solution may be found by using a surface coil, which is, in any case, always preferable for studies of the spinal cord. Intra- and extramedullary tumours can be diagnosed in the longitudinal plane, which is an advantage over CT. The spongiosa of the vertebrae is demonstrated easily and the intervertebral discs give a higher NMR signal (Fig. 108), making it possible to study degenerative lesions combined with cord or nerve root compression. Metastases of the vertebral bodies are seen well. NMR can replace diagnostic discography and, in many cases, myelography also. Whether this happens depends on the availability of the equipment and the cost of the examination.

Schematically, NMRI of the spine and contents can be shown as follows:

High signal intensity (bright)
high proton density
short T_1
long T_2

fat (subcutaneous, epidural, but also in lipomas)
  spongy bone
    nucleus pulposus of intervertebral disc
      spinal cord white matter ⎤   however, inversion of contrast
          grey matter ⎦⟶ with CSF with late SE sequence
     muscle
      CSF ——————————————⎦
        annulus fibrosus
         ligaments
          bone

        Low signal intensity (dark)
        low proton density
        long T_1
        short T_2

It is not clear whether NMRI can differentiate between granulation tissue and a residual part of a ruptured and prolapsed disc. It is also unclear whether NMR has advantages over CT in the diagnosis of malformations of the spine and its contents; especially the bony components of malformations, such as the bony spurs in diastematomyelia, or spondylolysis and spondylolisthesis may be demonstrated better by CT than by NMR.

III CARDIOVASCULAR SYSTEM

General remarks

NMR may be expected to make a valuable contribution in the diagnosis of a number of cardiovascular conditions; for example, aneurysm of the heart wall and ischaemic changes can be visualized. The advantage on CT is clear: because the blood is moving the magnetization in the vessels disappears, and therefore the chambers of the heart and the lumina of great vessels have a low signal intensity (black). Fourier analysis leads to fewer artefacts than the retrograde projection reconstruction method, so that, without gating, images of reasonable quality are obtained. However, for more detailed information it is necessary to collect the data exclusively at a selected point in the cardiac cycle, i.e., 'gating' (see Fig. 109). The heart is now 'at rest' and the image quality improves considerably.

In some of the illustrations (Fig. 110) the effect of gating (cardiac and respiratory) is clearly visible. There are many other possible applications of NMR in cardiovascular diagnosis. NMR has the potential to measure flow. A high flow leads to a loss of signal in the IR mode. With a slower flow the signal intensity increases. Eventually these data can be analysed quantitatively. Surface coils will not only improve the image quality, but also enable spectroscopy of the cardiac

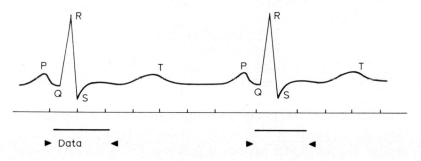

Figure 109. 'Gating' under electrocardiogram control. Data is only collected in a part of the cycle, in this case during the QRS period.

muscle to be performed. How important this will become clinically is not yet known.

Congenital heart disease

The previously mentioned possibility of obtaining contrast between the cardiac wall and the blood makes it possible to observe the muscles of the heart chambers and the large vessels. With the additional help of cardiac gating many congenital heart diseases can be visualized,

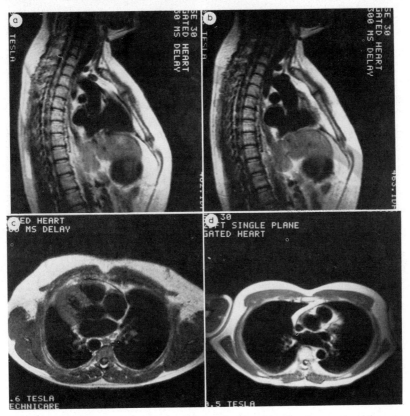

Figure 110. A series of NMR images made with cardiac gating with a 0.5 Tesla Technicare system. a, b, Sagittal sections through the chest. The chambers of the heart, the great vessels, diaphragm, liver and the thoracic vertebrae are seen well. c, d, Transverse sections with similar technique; c, at the level of the heart; d, at the level of the pulmonary arteries. The lung tissue has a low signal intensity. These images contain more information than those obtainable on third and fourth generation CT scanners.

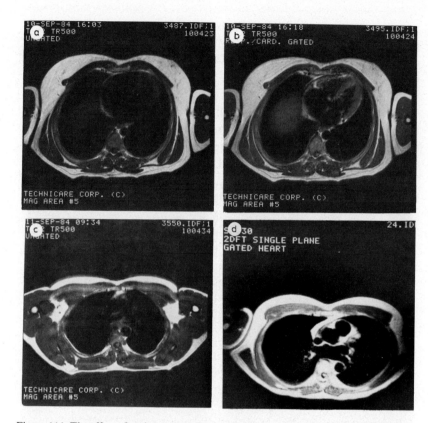

Figure 111. The effect of gating on imaging. a, Ungated image of the chest at the level of the heart. b, The same level in the same patient with both respiratory and cardiac gating. The improvement in information is convincing. c, d, Ungated and gated study at the level of the mediastinum.

e.g., atrical septal defect, ventricular septal defect, tricuspid valve atresia, stenosis of the aortic or mitral valve, transposition of the great vessels, persisting truncus arteriosus, etc. The many advantages of NMR are obvious in the preliminary orientating stages of the diagnosis. There is low energy radiation, and no contrast agents, no artefacts, good blood vessel wall separation, potential flow measurements, visualization of the heart muscle, etc.

Of course, it will often be necessary to complete thoracic studies with echocardiography and other more invasive diagnostic methods. The quality of NMR imaging is illustrated in Figures 110 and 111.

Experimental work has shown that the relaxation times in ischaemic areas lengthen. This process starts concurrently with the ischaemic condition and increases during the next 24 hours. This gives a potential for early detection. Under experimental conditions, and as has been shown with ECG gated studies (also in vivo), the ischaemic area in the heart muscle can be identified by SE pulse sequences because of the longer T_2. Phosphate compounds, such as adenosine triphosphate (ATP) and phosphocreatine, are essential to the metabolism of heart muscle. ^{31}P-NMR spectroscopy has the potential of obtaining information related to cardiac function. The differences between intra- and extracellular inorganic phosphate, indicating a change in pH, could be a delicate instrument in assessing local cardiac conditions. In that case, higher fields (2 Tesla) certainly are necessary, combined with the use of surface coils. The aim of such in vivo diagnosis clearly is to obtain spectrometic information from every pixel of the imaging field.

^{31}P-NMR spectroscopy could also indicate the efficiency of pharmacological treatment. Drugs could be compared in their effectiveness in the individual patient (see Ch. 8).

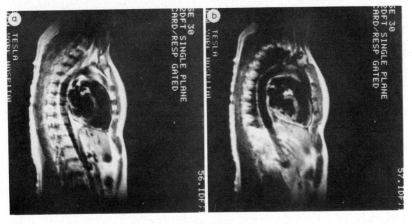

Figure 112. Oblique sagittal images of the chest and upper abdomen. a, b, Two oblique sagittal images in which the patient is turned to a left oblique position. Cardiac and respiratory gating were used. This position allows imaging of the thoracic and abdominal aorta.

Some of the illustrations (Figs. 111 and 112) are proof of the possibility of performing aortography with NMR. Aortic aneurysms can be seen without contrast injections. Flow measurements potentially are possible. Intramural thrombus formation can be seen, as well as 'fatty streaks' indicating early atheroma (or arteriosclerosis).

IV   INTERNAL ORGANS

General remarks

In imaging of the abdomen the possibility of obtaining NMR images in three dimensions without changing the patient's position is also of great importance. The cranio-caudad orientation of the blood vessels and the bilateral symmetry of the retroperitoneal organs already suggest that coronal images will give useful anatomic information. Transverse section is, of course, of importance in the upper abdomen, the liver and spleen and as an alternative image of the kidneys. Without contrast injection, the abdominal aorta and bifurcation and the vena cava can be seen. However, smaller vessels are observed equally well (the portal veins, the renal veins and arteries, the superior mesenteric artery, etc.). To visualize the bowels, one can consider letting the patient swallow sufficient water to obtain good contrast of the bowel. Of course, one may also consider other oral NMR contrast agents. Respiratory gating is mandatory for good quality images in the abdomen. Without this, the results in the mid-zone of the abdomen are disappointing.

Liver

The liver is seen on NMRI as a homogeneous organ of a moderate (grey) signal intensity with the usual pulse sequences. Blood vessels and widened biliary ducts are seen easily against this background. In many instances (Fig. 113) the portal venous system and the hepatic veins can be identified. In coronal slices the junction of the latter with the inferior vena cava can be seen (Fig. 114c). However, in this area

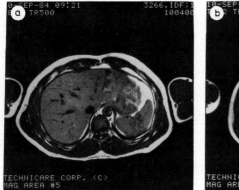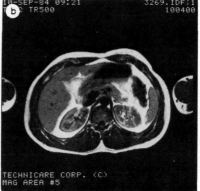

Figure 113. Sections through the upper abdomen. a, Section through liver and spleen. b, Section through the kidneys; clearly visible, surrounded by perirenal fat.

competition from much more cost-efficient ultrasound, which is versatile, and portable if need be, is clear. NMR has an advantage over CT, because Fourier analysis leads to fewer movement artefacts than the back projection technique used in CT systems. Of course, metastases, angiomas and primary tumours can be seen on NMR, as is usually the case with US and CT scans.

The role of NMR will probably be supplementary in those cases in which the other modalities give equivocal results. The near future will define better the positions of US, CT and NMR in respect to diagnosis in the upper abdomen. When NMRI is used as a primary diagnostic medium for the liver, then at least two pulse sequences have to be used, in order to lower the possibility of a false negative finding. It can be expected from the strong signal of fatty substances that NMRI may play a role in conditions in which there is an excessive storage of fat in the liver, as in fatty degeneration. This is also the case in pathological storage of iron. In the diagnosis of stones in the gallbladder NMR can be disappointing; US is superior. However, changes in the liquid contents of the gallbladder, indicative of function, are seen well on NMR.

Pancreas

With excellent imaging of the pancreas by CT and US there may be little need for NMR studies. Calcification is not seen as such on NMR

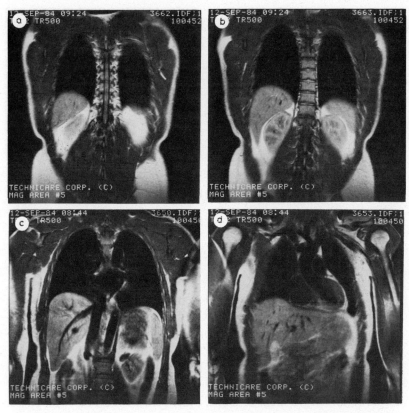

Figure 114. Coronal sections through chest and upper abdomen. a, Posteriorly in the chest the spinal canal is visible, and parts of the liver and spleen. b, Moving forwards, we find the kidneys, embedded in the perirenal fat. Good distinction between cortex and medulla. c, The larger vessels, aorta and vena cava are visible, as is the hepatic vein joining the inferior vena cava. d, The heart is depicted on this image with the aorta and pulmonary arteries.

images, which is a clear disadvantage. Certainly therefore, NMR will not be a first choice examination in pancreatic disease.

Kidneys and adrenals

Embedded in the perirenal fat, which has a high signal intensity, the kidneys can be seen extremely well on NMR: cortex and medulla are separated adequately (Fig. 113b). In coronal images, both kidneys, the ureters and retroperitoneal structures can be demonstrated in one image (Fig. 114); in transverse images, arteries and veins can be seen. Tumours, cysts and hydronephrosis are also demonstrated easily. Again, the question remains whether US scans are not capable of giving the same information at a much lower cost. Diseases of the renal parenchyma mostly demonstrate lengthening of T_1 and T_2. Tissue characterization in space-occupying lesions (malignant or benign) is not possible at this moment. The adrenals are also seen well on NMR images. One of the questions repeatedly asked of CT scans is whether it is possible to differentiate benign adrenal adenomas from metastases. It is still uncertain whether this differentiation can be made with sufficient authority by NMR.

V ABNORMALITIES IN THE PELVIS

The organs in the pelvis can be imaged on NMR without respiratory gating, because of the minimal movement in this area. Additionally, the sagittal images of bladder, rectum and genitals are very convincing, and add to the information obtained by CT and US. Of course, US has a place of its own in gynaecological diseases and in obstetrics.

VI MEDIASTINUM

NMRI of the mediastinum has clear advantages over CT and US. In NMR the blood vessels are seen with a dark lumen. Therefore, there is no need for a contrast injection to make the distinction between vascular and non-vascular structures (Fig. 114). Therefore, lymph glands can be located more easily. Thus far, however, it has not been possible to distinguish reactive lymph gland enlargement from malignant invasion. It has not been possible, to date, to distinguish sarcoidosis with enlargement of hilar lymph glands from reactive enlargement. Coronal, sagittal and axial slices can be made through the mediastinum, offering good detail of the bronchial tree, the pulmonary vessels, etc. (Fig. 115). Together with the mediastinum, lung tissue is imaged as a dark area (low signal intensity). Because of this low signal intensity abnormalities in the lung are easily demonstrable (Fig 116). Vascular disease of the mediastinum, e.g., an aortic aneurysm or retrosternal extension of the thyroid gland, can be seen easily.

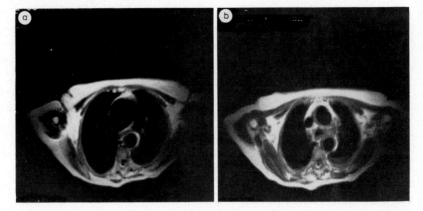

Figure 115. Images of a patient with an aorta aneurysm. a, b, These images were obtained without cardiac and respiratory gating on a 0.5 Tesla system (Technicare).

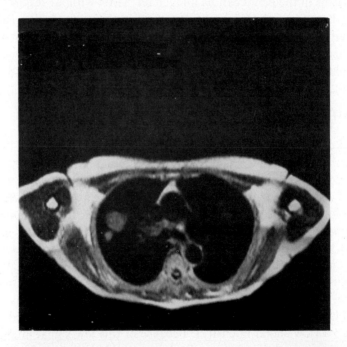

Figure 116. Because of the low signal intensity, tumours in the lung parenchyma are detected easily. In this case, a lesion in the right lung with a satellite and an enlarged lymph node in the hilus is shown.

Some experiences have been reported regarding NMR studies of the hips (Fig. 117), knees, osteosarcomas of the limbs, etc. The last category is especially interesting because it gives information that is not available by other means, i.e., the exact extension of the process inside and outside the bone. Examination of the muscles is very rewarding in small-bore magnets with stronger magnetic fields, so that spectroscopy can be performed, e.g., ^{31}P examinations (see Ch. 8).

VIII MISCELLANEOUS

The use of surface coils and contrast agents will make it necessary to re-evaluate many of the diagnostic algorithms. This will certainly be true for the orbit, the petrous bone, the thyroid, the spine, the heart, etc. Therefore, it is impossible to estimate even roughly the role of NMRI in diagnostic radiology in the next decade.

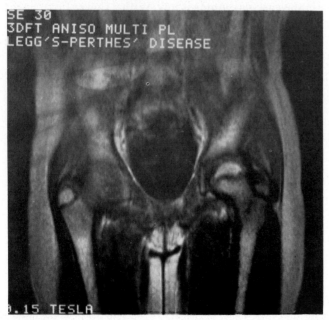

Figure 117. Example of an NMR image in disease of the hip (morbus perthes). This image was made on a 0.15 Tesla system (Technicare).

In 1959 Singer demonstrated the possibility of measuring flow in a tube using an NMR signal. The first experiments were performed on the tails of mice (Fig. 118) placed with a transmitter and receiver coil in a static magnetic field. The NMR signal changed with the velocity of the blood flow in the tail artery. This experiment was applied, rather unexpectedly, to measuring the flow of kerosine in the tubes of rocket engines without placing any measuring device in the stream itself. This proved to be a simple task, because these tubes possessed a constant diameter, so that the velocity had only to be multiplied by the surface area of the lumen. The principle of flow measurement is simple. With an RF transmitter a 180° or 90° pulse is given. Thus, a bolus with labeled protons is obtained which changes position with flow. Therefore, the signal in the receiving coil will also change, and this change will depend on the flow velocity. It had already been noted in imaging techniques that when blood flows away from the examined slice and is replaced by blood that has not undergone the RF pulse, the signal intensity in the vascular lumen is low. With a slower flow the intensity of the signal increases. In imaging techniques this can give an impression of the flow velocity. However, this phenomenon is difficult to quantitate. With cardiac gating it is possible to relate the signal of the blood, e.g., in the thoracic aorta, to a certain phase of the cardiac cycle. One image can be obtained with maximal flow (systole), another one

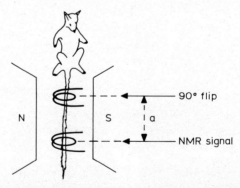

Figure 118. The 'Singer' experiment to measure flow. After the 90° pulse it takes x mseconds for the NMR signal to change. To measure the flow, the distance, time, diameter of the tube (vessel) and intensity of the change in the NMR signal are necessary.

with minimal flow (diastole). This can also give a qualitative indication of flow.

In imaging a volume, T_1 may be shortened because blood which has responded to the initial pulse flows out of the volume. In principle, this gives a possibility for estimating regional blood flow. The influence of flow on the signal intensity is also dependent on the chosen pulse sequence. In the SR sequence (Fig. 119), increase in blood flow may lead to a higher signal intensity. After the initial 90° pulse the magne-

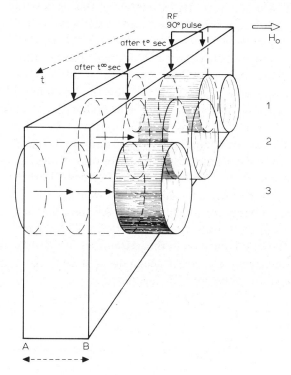

Figure 119. NMR signal and flow. In the figure a situation is shown in which the layer A–B is selectively irradiated with a 90° pulse of narrow band width. Immediately after the pulse, the situation in the blood vessels, which lie perpendicular to the selected layer, is illustrated at number 1. The protons are nutated through 90° and there is no magnetization along the z-axis. If after t^0 mseconds a measuring pulse is given, a fraction of the irradiated protons has disappeared from the layer, and is replaced by protons that still possess a full magnetization along the z-axis (2). If a longer interpulse time is chosen (t^∞) or if the flow is faster, even more of the irradiated protons will have disappeared from the layer and will be replaced by protons still having the full magnetization, M_z.
Therefore, the signal intensity increases.

tization along the x-axis is zero. A 90° RF read pulse, given shortly after the first pulse, would show, in the absence of flow, a low value of magnetization along the x-axis. In the presence of flow this blood will stream away from the slice and be replaced by blood that has not been exposed to the 90° pulse. A read pulse at this time will find a large M_z, and therefore the signal intensity is also high. The faster the flow, the higher the signal intensity. It is clear that there is a quantitative relationship between the velocity of flow (F_v) and the t_i and t_r of the pulse sequence. Therefore, accurate estimation of flow is possible.

Of course, the spin echo sequence can also be used. Following the initial 90° pulse, after t_i mseconds a refocussing pulse (180°) is given. It will be evident that only those protons which were submitted to the first (90°) pulse and are still present in the irradiated layer will respond with a spin echo. The faster the flow the less intense the NMR signal will be. The slower the flow, the higher the intensity of the NMR signal. Here also, there is a quantitative relation between the flow velocity, the t_i, the t_e and the t_r of the pulse sequence. In spin echo measurement molecular diffusion is also of importance. In the future, flow measurements in vivo by NMR will be developed further. This will help to obtain information about the flow in coronary arteries and in bypasses, probably with the use of surface coils. Surface coils could also be used to quantitate flow in the brain. The effect of vascular surgery of the brain and also in the extremities probably will be measured non-invasively by NMR techniques. It could be that special equipment will be developed for this purpose.

NMR spectroscopy in vivo

8

I   INTRODUCTION

Although this book deals mainly with NMR imaging techniques, this chapter will review some elementary aspects of NMR spectroscopy in vivo, because this has already demonstrated a certain clinical value. From this discussion it will become clear what conditions have to be satisfied to obtain spectroscopic information from biological systems.

Of the nuclei that are of biological importance and which have a magnetic moment, ^{31}P (natural abundance, 100%), ^{23}Na (100%), ^{13}C (1.1%) and ^{14}N (99.6%) are the most interesting, because of their involvement in biochemical processes. None of these nuclei approach the numerical density of hydrogen atoms in living tissue. Also, their sensitivity for NMR is less than that of protons. A propos of this, one may speak of the 'receptivity' of nuclei, which is the product of natural abundance and sensitivity. Therefore, these nuclei are less fitted for NMR imaging techniques: the signal becomes weaker unless the volume of the voxels is increased.

Given a nucleus in the examined organ with a concentration of 0.01 to that of protons and a 0.1 sensitivity to that of protons, the receptivity of that nucleus would be 0.001. This means that for an equal signal to noise ratio (S/N) the voxel size would have to be 1 cm^3 instead of 1 mm^3. The question arises as to whether information obtained from voxels of this size can give relevant clinical information. On the other hand, we also have to take into consideration the possible repetition rates of the pulse sequences. ^{23}Na, for instance, has a very short T_1, making a high repetition rate possible. Even with a low receptivity a satisfactory S/N can be obtained within a reasonable time limit.

In NMR spectroscopy the goal is not to obtain images, but spectra in which the chemical shifts of the various nuclear spins have been resolved. For ^{31}P spectra these could be the shifts of the α, β and γ nuclei in adenosine triphosphate and other phosphorus compounds. To resolve these chemical shifts a reasonably good field homogeneity is necessary (of the order of 1:10^6). Usually, the homogeneity of whole-body magnets is not adequate, being of the order of 1:10^5; also the sensitivity of ^{31}P at field strengths of 1–2 Tesla is only moderate.

These spectra can be measured more adequately at higher field strengths. A good field homogeneity with good S/N are achieved in narrow-bore, high-field magnets. Most of the spectroscopic results now available have been obtained in laboratory experiments with animals, and perfused organs in cryomagnetic systems with bores varying from 3 to 30 cm. If the bore permits an arm or a leg to be put in the magnet, ^{31}P spectroscopy of human muscles is possible. From these experiments it has become clear that such information can be of great clinical importance. One can expect that spectroscopic studies gradually will be performed in whole-body systems with higher field strength, or via surface coils with better S/N and improved local homogeneity. Some of this 'work in progress' has been published recently.

II ^{31}P-NMR SPECTROSCOPY

The role of phosphorus in the metabolism in the human body is well known, especially of compounds such as phosphocreatine, adenosine triphosphate (ATP), adenosine diphosphate (ADP) and inorganic phosphorus, the latter both intra- and extracellular (Fig. 120). Tiny

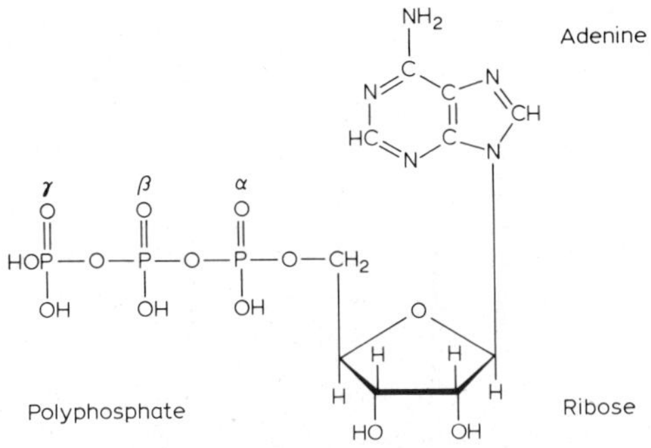

Figure 120. The structure of adenosine triphosphate (ATP). During the transformation into adenosine diphosphate (ADP), energy is liberated, which serves as an energy source for cell metabolism of the tissue. The structure of the Mg-ATP complex is not known fully. It is thought that the Mg^{2+} interacts mainly with the oxygen atoms.

shifts in the resonance frequency of the phosphorus nucleus (chemical shifts) come into existence because the magnetic field of the magnet is shielded by electrons in its vicinity.

These shifts are an order greater than in the case of protons, and therefore can be measured more easily. A field homogeneity of $1:10^6$ is sufficient to resolve these shifts.

In ischaemic conditions, the so-called oxidative phosphorylation is blocked, and ADP cannot be transformed into ATP to reload the energy source of the tissue. Phosphocreatine, which normally provides a rapid way of donating a high-energy phosphate link, is used up rapidly under these conditions and its concentration decreases (Fig. 123).

The system now has to rely on the much less efficient process of anaerobic glycolysis, in which lactic acid is produced, with a subsequent lowering of the pH (e.g., from 7.2 to 6.5). The lower pH causes the intracellular phosphorus to increase. The chemical shift of this inorganic phosphorus can be used spectroscopically to estimate the pH. If conditions return to normal, then the speed at which the prevailing conditions return depend on the condition of the tissue.

Two aspects have become clear, especially with regard to ischaemic changes in heart muscle. In the first place, it is possible to assess local areas of the organ; the severity of an ischaemic condition can be estimated. Secondly, these data open up a method of examining the effect of pharmacological substances protecting tissue against oxygen deprivation. Non-invasive pharmacology in vivo is possible in this way.

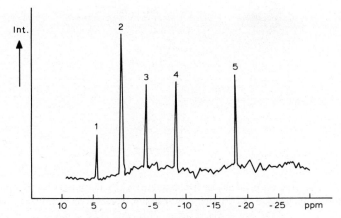

Figure 121. ^{31}P-NMR spectrum of tissue under normal conditions in vivo. 1, Inorganic phosphorus; 2, phosphocreatine; 3–5, ATP.

The ^{31}P-NMR spectrum in vivo has five characteristic resonances (Fig. 121): 1. Inorganic phosphorus – the chemical shift is pH dependent. 2. Phosphocreatine, the chemical shift is constant and can be used as a point of reference, from which the other shifts can be measured. 3. The γ resonance of ATP. 4. The α resonance of ATP. 5. The β resonance of ATP.

Inorganic phosphorus demonstrates two relatively weak resonances, originating from ^{31}P within and outside the cells. Their chemical shifts are different, because the intra- and extracellular pH is

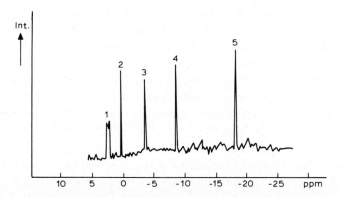

Figure 122. ^{31}P spectrum following ischaemia. The phosphocreatine signal (2) has decreased; the peak of inorganic phosphorus has shifted towards the phosphocreatine (1→2), indicating a fall in the pH; the ATP signals have hardly changed.

different. This susceptibility to pH changes is caused by ionizable H^+ atoms in inorganic phosphorus. Intra- and extracellular pH can be measured in this way. If the pH decreases, the resonance of the inorganic phosphorus shifts in the direction of phosphocreatine. This shift can be measured accurately. The intensity of the signals is proportional to the concentration of the substance causing it, so that quantitative measurements are possible. Experimentally, one can study the changes brought about by ischaemic conditions (see Figs. 122 and 123). Changes to be expected are: lowering of the pH, decrease of the phosphocreatine concentration, increase of the glyco-phosphates, and some decrease in the amount of ATP

Other abnormalities in phosphorus metabolism can be studied in the same way. It has been reported that ^{31}P-NMR spectroscopy can reveal information about the viability of transplant organs, e.g., kidneys, by measuring the intracellular pH. ^{31}P-NMR spectroscopy has also been used in studies of tumour malignancy in which the changes

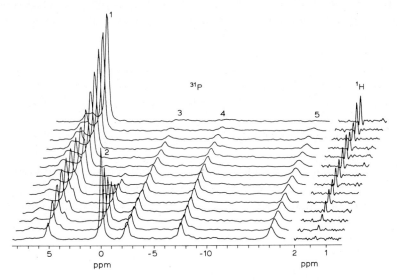

Figure 123. ^{31}P and ^{1}H spectra of a leg muscle of a rat, immediately after removal, and subsequently repeated at hourly intervals. The spectra on the left are ^{31}P spectra, measured at 101.2 MHz; the spectra on the right are ^{1}H spectra, obtained at 250 MHz. The ischaemic changes are shown well in the ^{31}P spectra. Phosphocreatine (2) and, to a lesser extent, ATP (3,4,5) decrease. Inorganic phosphorus (1) increases. The resonance in the ^{1}H spectra originates from lactate acid. (By courtesy of J. Bulthuis and P.A. Huyning, Free University, Amsterdam, and J.A.B. Lohman, Bruker Physik.)

in pH have been studied after glucose loading, the so-called Warburg effect. This is especially obvious in fast-growing tumours. It is an example of an impetus to the NMR analysis of specific tumour behaviour. It is obvious that ^{31}P-NMR spectroscopy can be used to study fundamental biological processes. With improvement of the whole-body systems, ^{31}P-NMR spectroscopy might become of great importance in oncology. With equipment in which an arm or leg can be inserted, it is already possible at present to examine the influence of muscle exercise on the ^{31}P spectrum. This could be important in the study of programmes for training and rehabilitation. One disease from the series of muscle dystrophies can already be identified by way of ^{31}P-NMR spectroscopy – McArdle's disease. In this disease there exists an inborn error of metabolism, with a deficiency of glycogen phosphorylase. Before ^{31}P-NMR spectroscopy allowed a definitive diagnosis, this could only be obtained by a biopsy, demonstrating an excess of glycogen and a shortage of phosphorylase. ^{31}P-NMR spectroscopy shows that after exercise no lowering of pH takes place, and that the concentration of phospocreatine does not decrease. This points to the absence of lactate production.

In the training of athletes this non-invasive technique might be used to assess the efficacy of training schedules, especially the restoration of normal levels of phosphorus compounds after exercise.

III ^{23}Na SPECTROSCOPY

Sodium also plays an important role in biological processes. Examples are the active transportation of substances such as glucose, and the build-up of action potentials along nerve fibres. In these cases the basic biological mechanism is the so-called sodium-potassium (Fig. 124) or ion pump. This is fundamental in the transport of molecules through the membranes of tissue cells. This transport occurs against the direction of concentration and electrical gradients. ^{23}Na$^+$ is present extracellularly in higher concentrations than intracellularly (142:10 mmol/l), whereas for K$^+$ the reverse is true (5:190 mmol/l). The transport of sodium through the cell membrane, against this gradient, demands energy. This is provided by the ATP–ADP transformation in the mitochondria of the cells: ATP $\rightarrow$ ADP + P$_i$ + E (P$_i$ = inorganic phosphor, E = energy).

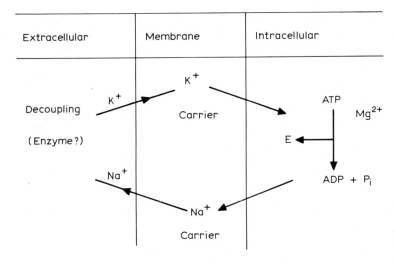

Figure 124. Schematic representation of the sodium-potassium pump. ATP serves as energy donor and makes the system oxygen dependent.

[23]Na is present in the brain in higher concentrations than in the rest of the body, e.g., twice as much as in muscle. The resonance frequency at 1 Tesla is about 10 MHz. The NMR sensitivity is $9.25 \cdot 10^{-2}$: about 0.1 of the sensitivity of protons. What may be of importance in future research is that in ischaemic processes the intracellular amount of [23]Na increases.

Probably this is a very early effect, measurable within hours from the onset of ischaemia. Whether it is of clinical importance remains to be seen. Another important point may be the higher concentration of [23]Na in malignant tumours. Perhaps this presents an opportunity to differentiate relatively 'benign' from 'malignant' growth. With 1.5–2 Tesla systems it is already possible to obtain this kind of information in brain tumours, although the S/N of the spectra is far from excellent.

IV OTHER NUCLEI

Other nuclei that are of potential interest for NMR spectroscopy in vivo are [14]N (99.63%), [19]F (100%), [17]O (3.7%) and [13]C (1.108%). For their use in NMR spectroscopy in vivo, special problems have to be solved, e.g., the low sensitivity for NMR at the low concentration in human tissues. The future will tell in which cases these problems can be solved and whether the information so obtained is clinically relevant.

Biological side effects

9

Three components of the NMR imaging system are of importance with regard to biological side effects, namely, the static magnetic field, the time-dependent field gradients and the radiofrequency pulses. Extensive research has shown that no deleterious side effects attributed to NMR imaging may be expected. These investigations may be studied in the publications of Budinger (1982) and Mansfield and Morris (1983). We will discuss briefly the three above-mentioned components.

The magnetic field exerts a force on all ferromagnetic elements in the body, e.g., metallic implants, protheses, clips, etc. Electric current-dependent equipment, such as pacemakers, can be influenced by the field because of the Lorentz force the field exerts on moving charges.

Non-static field gradients can induce currents in the body. The human body contains numerous ions and may be looked upon as a conductor. In accordance with Faraday's laws of induction, a changing magnetic field induces a current in a conductor. Switching the field gradients on and off will indeed induce an electric current in tissues.

The radiofrequency radiation penetrates the body. Interaction will occur between the electric component of the radiation and the electric dipoles in the tissue, e.g., the water molecules. The resulting heat dissipated depends on the frequency of the radiation. The frequencies used in NMR imaging (10–60 MHz) certainly cause heating of the tissues, dependent also on the intensity of the RF pulses. Increasing the magnetic field strength, necessitating higher RF frequencies, will also increase heat dissipation. These effects are analogous to the heating in magnetron ovens and in diathermy.

Influence on the conduction of electric potentials along nerve fibres and the electroencephalogram cannot be ruled out theoretically. However, experiments have demonstrated that these effects are negligible or even immeasurable with the field strengths and energies currently in use. Genetic damage has not been demonstrated.

Certain safety guidelines can be derived from the foregoing discussion: ferromagnetic implants in the body, such as some of the metal clips used in the treatment of aneurysms, will react to the field forces, with possible complications. Large metallic protheses can be heated up to too high a level. Pacemakers can be de-regulated because of the static field and the time-dependent field gradients. Patients with such a risk factor must be examined by imaging methods other than NMRI. The changing field gradients could have an exciting influence on the cerebral nervous system, a possible risk factor in patients with epilepsy. However, we have examined patients with epilepsy without any clinical or EEG changes. The field gradients eventually could interfere with the heart action, and lead to ventricular fibrillation. The induced current intensity in NMRI systems, however, lies at least two magnitudes below the threshold of these biological effects. The National Radiological Protection Board of the United Kingdom has published the following safety guidelines: field strength, maximal 2.5 Tesla; field gradients, < 20 T sec^{-1} maximal alternating frequency ($\geqq 10$ mseconds); RF pulses, maximal 15 MHz, <1 W/kG absorbed power.

At this moment there is already experience with static magnetic fields of up to 2.5 Tesla (> 100 MHz) for whole-body imaging. Therefore, the safety guidelines will have to be adapted. All available data show a broad margin between the applied magnetic forces and energies and the thresholds for hazardous biological interactions. In practice, therefore, the precautions are only valid for the aforementioned groups, i.e., patients with metallic implants and large protheses of ferromagnetic material, and patients with pacemakers. Apart from these limitations, the problem of inaccessibility of patients during the examination remains. It is difficult to provide critically ill patients with 'life support' systems.

Seriously ill patients, premature children, etc., cannot be examined by NMR unless further technical developments eliminate this problem.

Appendix I

10

VECTORS

Vectors are very important in NMR: the magnetization of a sample, the static field and the RF field are all vectors. In the following we shall discuss some concepts of vector calculus.

A vector is characterized by its magnitude and direction. A simple example is the 'position vector', $\vec{r}$, with components x, y, z. The length of $\vec{r}$, denoted by r, is given by

$$r = \sqrt{x^2 + y^2 + z^2}$$

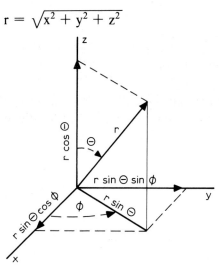

Figure 125

The direction of $\vec{r}$ can be defined with the angles θ and ø (Fig. 125). One has: x = r sin

154 $\theta \cos \phi$ y = r $\sin \theta \sin \phi$, z = r $\cos \theta$.

Analogously, the magnetization vector $\vec{M}$ has components M_x, M_y and M_z. Its length M is given by

$$M = \sqrt{M_x^2 + M_y^2 + M_z^2}$$

The components are: $M_x = M \sin \theta \cos \phi$, $M_y = M \sin \theta \sin \phi$, $M_z = |M \cos \theta$ (Fig. 126).

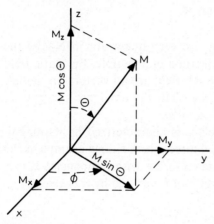

Figure 126

Addition of vectors

We first define three unit vectors: $\vec{e}_x, \vec{e}_y, \vec{e}_z$; they are directed along the positive x-, y- and z-axes and their lengths are unity. A general vector $\vec{a}$

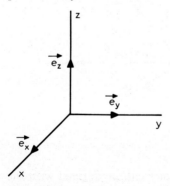

Figure 127

with components a_x, a_y, a_z can be expressed in the three unit vectors

$$\vec{a} = a_x\vec{e}_x + a_y\vec{e}_y + a_z\vec{e}_z$$

The sum of two vectors, $\vec{a} + \vec{b}$, in which

$$\vec{b} = b_x\vec{e}_x + b_y\vec{e}_y + b_z\vec{e}_z$$

is defined as

$$\vec{a} + \vec{b} = (a_x + b_x)\vec{e}_x + (a_y + b_y)\vec{e}_y + (a_z + b_z)\vec{e}_z$$

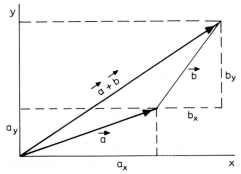

Figure 128

This definition expresses the 'parallelogram rule', as illustrated in Figure 128 for the two-dimensional case. The vectors $\vec{a}$ and $\vec{b}$ are 'free' vectors, which may be displaced with retention of direction.

The difference between two vectors $\vec{a}$ and $\vec{b}$ is defined analogously

$$\vec{a} - \vec{b} = (a_x - b_x)\vec{e}_x + (a_y - b_y)\vec{e}_y + (a_z - b_z)\vec{e}_z.$$

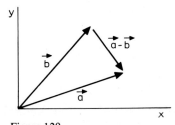

Figure 129

156 The difference vector $\vec{a} - \vec{b}$ goes from the endpoint of $\vec{b}$ to the endpoint of $\vec{a}$. Addition and subtraction of more than two vectors is defined by extension of the given definitions.

Multiplication of vectors

The simplest case is multiplication of a vector by a scalar, i.e., a number. If the vector is denoted by $\vec{a}$ and the scalar c, the product is

$$c\vec{a} = (ca_x)\vec{e}_x + (ca_y)\vec{e}_y + (ca_z)\vec{e}_z$$

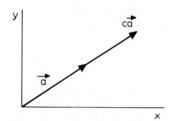

Figure 130

If c is positive, the product vector is parallel to $\vec{a}$; if c = 0, the null vector is generated; for negative c the product vector is antiparallel to $\vec{a}$. There are two possible definitions of the product of a vector and another vector: the 'internal' or 'scalar' product and the 'external' or 'cross' product. In order to distinguish the two products, two multiplication symbols are introduced. The scalar product of two vectors $\vec{a}$ and $\vec{b}$ is denoted by $\vec{a} \cdot \vec{b}$, the cross product by $\vec{a} \times \vec{b}$.

The scalar product is by definition

$$\vec{a} \cdot \vec{b} = a\,b\,\cos\theta$$

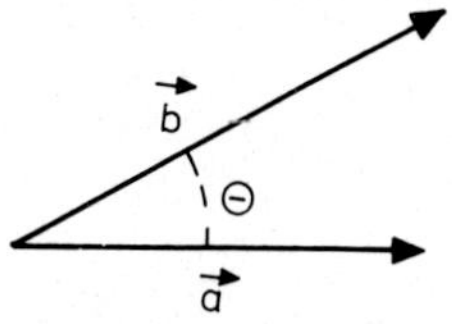

Figure 131

The product is a number: the product of the lengths of the vectors times the cosine of the angle. The scalar product of two perpendicular

vectors is zero. An application of the scalar product is the concept
'mechanical work': the work (dA) by a force ($\vec{F}$) done over a distance
($\vec{dr}$) is given by: $dA = \vec{F} \cdot \vec{dr}$. The work is a scalar, obtained as the
scalar product of two vectors.

Without proof we give the relation

$$\vec{a} \cdot \vec{b} = a_x b_x + a_y b_y + a_z b_z$$

The numerical value of a scalar product can be obtained directly from
the components of the vectors.

The cross product of two vectors $\vec{a}$ and $\vec{b}$ generates a new vector,
which by definition is perpendicular to $\vec{a}$ and $\vec{b}$ and whose length is the
product of a and b times the sine of the enclosed angle: $a\,b\,\sin\theta$. To fix
the direction of the product vector $\vec{a} \times \vec{b}$ unambiguously, the screw
rule is adopted: turn $\vec{a}$ towards $\vec{b}$; the direction of $\vec{a} \times \vec{b}$ coincides with
that of the screw. The cross products of the three unit vectors are very
simple

$$\vec{e}_x \times \vec{e}_x = \vec{e}_y \times \vec{e}_y = \vec{e}_z \times \vec{e}_z = 0$$

$$\vec{e}_x \times \vec{e}_y = \vec{e}_z; \quad \vec{e}_y \times \vec{e}_z = \vec{e}_x; \quad \vec{e}_z \times \vec{e}_x = \vec{e}_y$$

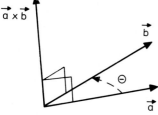

Figure 132

The former relations follow from $\sin 0° = 0$; the latter from $\sin 90° = 1$.

The commutative property does not hold

$$\vec{e}_x \times \vec{e}_y = -(\vec{e}_y \times \vec{e}_x)$$

$$\vec{a} \times \vec{b} = -(\vec{b} \times \vec{a})$$

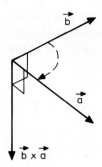

Figure 133

The cross product can be developed

$$\vec{a} \times \vec{b} = [a_x\vec{e}_x + a_y\vec{e}_y + a_z\vec{e}_z] \times [b_x\vec{e}_x + b_y\vec{e}_y + b_z\vec{e}_z]$$
$$= (a_yb_z - b_za_y)\vec{e}_x + (a_zb_x - a_xb_z)\vec{e}_y + (a_xb_y - a_yb_x)\vec{e}_z$$

An illustration of the cross product is the torque $\vec{\tau}$ exerted on the magnetization $\vec{M}$ by a magnetic field $\vec{H}_0$:

$$\vec{\tau} = \vec{M} \times \vec{H}_0$$

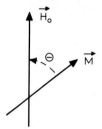

Figure 134

The torque $\vec{\tau}$ is perpendicular to $\vec{M}$ and $\vec{H}_0$ and has length $MH_0 \sin \theta$. The magnetization $\vec{M}$ can be viewed as a dipole: when $\vec{M}$ is parallel to the field, the torque is zero, as implied by $\sin 0° = 0$.

A further illustration is the angular momentum $\vec{L}$ of a particle; it is defined by

$$\vec{L} = \vec{r} \times \vec{p} = m\vec{r} \times \vec{v}$$

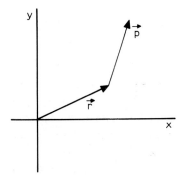

Figure 135

$\vec{r}$ is the position vector, m its mass and $\vec{v}$ its velocity. If the particle describes a circular path: L = mvR, a relation used in chapter 2.

Another relation used is $(d/dt)\,\vec{L} = \vec{\tau}$, in which $\vec{\tau}$ is the torque. For a single particle the torque is defined by $\vec{\tau} = \vec{r} \times \vec{F}$; $\vec{F}$ is the force on the particle. To prove the above relation, differentiate $\vec{L}$ with respect to t

$$\frac{d\vec{L}}{dt} = m\,[\vec{r} \times \frac{d\vec{v}}{dt} + \frac{d\vec{r}}{dt} \times \vec{v}]$$

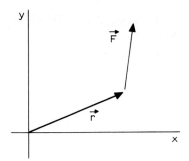

Figure 136

Since $(d\vec{r}/dt) = \vec{v}$ by definition, the second term on the right vanishes; introducing $\vec{F} = m(d\vec{v}/dt)$ completes the proof: $(d\vec{L}/dt) = \vec{\tau}$.

For more details about physical applications of vectors the reader is referred to M. Alonso and E.J. Finn, Fundamental University Physics, Addison-Wesley Publishing Company Inc., Reading, MA, U.S.A.

Appendix 2

PROOF OF THE RELATION $n_+ - n_- = \dfrac{N}{2} \left(\dfrac{\Delta E}{kT}\right) (1 - e^{-t/T_1})$

Consider a sample with N nuclear spins which are distributed over two energy levels. The occupation numbers are n_+ and n_-. The energy difference between the levels is $\Delta E = \gamma (h/2\pi) H_0$.

The sample was placed in the field at time $t = 0$; then $n_+ = n_-$ in accordance with the above relation. For large t the exponential is close to zero and the relation predicts that the equilibrium distribution is such that $(n_+ - n_-) = (N/2) \cdot (\Delta E/kT)$. To verify this consider Boltzmann's distribution law: $(n_+/n_-) = e^{\Delta E/kT}$. For small $\Delta E/kT$, the exponential can be approximated:

$$e^{\Delta E/kT} = 1 + \frac{\Delta E}{kT}$$

from which, after substitution

$$n_+ - n_- = n_- \left(\frac{\Delta E}{kT}\right) \simeq \frac{N}{2} \left(\frac{\Delta E}{kT}\right)$$

To prove the general expression, we introduce transition probabilities per second W_{+-} and W_{-+}. Detailed balancing requires

$$\frac{d}{dt} n_+ = -W_{+-}n_+ + W_{-+}n_-$$

$$\frac{d}{dt} n_- = +W_{+-}n_+ - W_{-+}n_-$$

from which

$$\frac{d}{dt} (n_+ - n_-) = -2 (W_{+-} n_+ - W_{-+} n_-)$$

In thermodynamic equilibrium the left hand side is zero; hence,

$$\frac{n_+}{n_-} = \frac{W_{-+}}{W_{+-}} = 1 + \frac{\Delta E}{kT}$$

As expected, the relaxation process W_{-+} is somewhat longer than W_{+-}. Introducing the mean transition probability $W = \frac{1}{2}(W_{+-} + W_{-+})$, we have

$$W_{+-} = W(1 - \frac{\Delta E}{2kT})$$

$$W_{-+} = W(1 + \frac{\Delta E}{2kT})$$

After substitution

$$\frac{d}{dT}(n_+ - n_-) = -2W[(n_+ - n_-) - \frac{N}{2}(\frac{\Delta E}{kT})].$$

Inspection shows that this differential equation is satisfied by

$$n_+ - n_- = \frac{N}{2}(\frac{\Delta E}{kT})(1 - e^{-2Wt})$$

Equating 2W to the reciprocal relaxation time T_1 gives the relation to be proven. The factor 2 reflects the fact that reversal of one spin, changes the difference in occupation number by two.

Appendix 3

LARMOR'S THEOREM

According to Larmor's theorem, the magnetization $\vec{M}$ precesses about the field $\vec{H}_0$ with the 'Larmor frequency', $\omega_L = \gamma H_0$.

To prove this relation we start with the well-known formula from classical mechanics (see Appendix 1)

$$\vec{\tau} = \frac{d}{dt} \vec{L}$$

$\vec{L}$ is the angular momentum of the nuclear spin system, obtained by summing up vectorially the angular momenta of the separate spins. The magnetic moment of this ensemble is $\vec{M} = \gamma \vec{L}$, in which γ is the gyromagnetic ratio.

The magnetic field $\vec{H}_0$ exerts a torque on the magnetization of magnitude and direction given by $(\vec{M} \times \vec{H}_0)$. Note that the cross denotes external vector multiplication (see Appendix 1):

$$\vec{M} \times \vec{H}_0 = (M_y H_{0z} - M_z H_{0y}) \vec{e}_x +$$

$$(M_z H_{0x} - M_x H_{0z}) \vec{e}_y + (M_x H_{0y} - M_y H_{0x}) \vec{e}_z.$$

($M_{x,y,z}$ are the components of $\vec{M}$ along the axes x,y,z of the reference frame; $H_{0x,0y,0z}$ those of $\vec{H}_0$ and $\vec{e}_{x,y,z}$ are unit vectors along the axes.)

The 'equation of motion' for the magnetization is

$$\frac{d}{dt} \vec{M} = \gamma \vec{M} \times \vec{H}_0$$

Written out in the three components

$$\frac{dM_x}{dt} = \gamma(M_y H_{0z} - M_z H_{0y})$$

$$\frac{dM_y}{dt} = \gamma(M_z H_{0x} - M_x H_{0z})$$

$$\frac{dM_z}{dt} = \gamma(M_x H_{0y} - M_y H_{0x})$$

For simplicity and without loss of generality, we choose the direction of the static field along the z-axis of the frame of reference; then H_{0x} = H_{0y} = 0; H_{0z} = H_0. The three equations simplify to

$$\frac{dM_x}{dt} = \gamma H_0 M_y$$

$$\frac{dM_y}{dt} = -\gamma H_0 M_x$$

$$\frac{dM_z}{dt} = 0$$

The third equation means that M_z is constant in time, as expected for a precession about the z-axis. The two remaining equations are satisfied by

$$M_x = M_{tr} \cos \omega_L t$$

$$M_y = -M_{tr} \sin \omega_L t$$

with $\omega_L = \gamma H_0$, as is readily verifiable. The transverse component of the magnetization, rotating with constant angular velocity about H_0, is

$$M_{tr} = \sqrt{M_x^2 + M_y^2}.$$

Appendix 4

THE EQUIVALENCE OF A LINEARLY POLARIZED ALTERNATING FIELD AND TWO COUNTER-ROTATING FIELDS

An alternating field polarized along the x-axis with frequency ω and amplitude $2H_1$ can be written as $H_x = 2H_1 \cos \omega t$.

The two rotating fields which, after superposition, give the linear field are

$H_x = H_1 \cos \omega t$ $\qquad\qquad\qquad$ $H_x = H_1 \cos \omega t$

and

$H_y = H_1 \sin \omega t$ $\qquad\qquad\qquad$ $H_y = -H_1 \sin \omega t$

The left field rotates counterclockwise, the right field clockwise (Fig. 137). To verify this, start from $t = 0$ so that $H_x = H_1$; $H_y = 0$; for small t one has $H_y > 0$ (left) and $H_y < 0$ (right). The sense of the rotation is then established. The amplitudes of the two rotating fields are equal: $H_x^2 + H_y^2 = H_1^2$. In connection with energy dissipation in the form of heat, only one of the two components is generated in modern spectrometers. This is of importance in high-field, high-frequency imaging equipment.

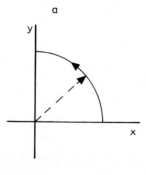
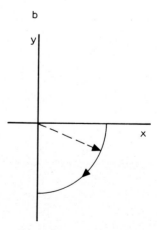

Figure 137

Appendix 5

THE ROTATING FRAME

It has been shown in Appendix 3 that the time dependence of the magnetization, under the influence of a magnetic field $\vec{H}$, the vector sum of the static field $\vec{H}_0$ and the rotating field $\vec{H}_1$, can now be written as

$$\frac{dM_x}{dt} = \gamma(M_y H_z - M_z H_y)$$

$$\frac{dM_y}{dt} = \gamma(M_z H_x - M_x H_z)$$

$$\frac{dM_z}{dt} = \gamma(M_x H_y - M_y H_x)$$

The static field is again chosen along the z-axis ($H_{0x} = H_{0y} = 0$; $H_{0z} = H_0$), the rotating field in the transversal plane ($H_x = H_1 \cos \omega t$, $H_y = -H_1 \sin \omega t$). Substitution gives

$$\frac{dM_x}{dt} = \gamma H_0 M_y + \gamma H_1 \sin \omega t \, M_z$$

$$\frac{dM_y}{dt} = \gamma H_1 \cos \omega t \, M_z - \gamma H_0 M_x$$

$$\frac{dM_z}{dt} = -\gamma H_1 \sin \omega t \, M_x - \gamma H_1 \cos \omega t \, M_y$$

On the right, the quantities γH_0 (i.e., the Larmor frequency) and γH_1 are found. The latter quantity also has the dimension of frequency; for brevity we introduce $\gamma H_1 = \omega_1$. The frequency ω_1 characterizes the amplitude of the RF field, ω its frequency. After substitution

$$\frac{dM_x}{dt} = \omega_L M_y + \omega_1 \sin \omega t \, M_z$$

$$\frac{dM_y}{dt} = \omega_1 \cos \omega t \, M_z - \omega_L M_x$$

$$\frac{dM_z}{dt} = -\omega_1 \sin \omega t \, M_x - \omega_1 \cos \omega t \, M_y$$

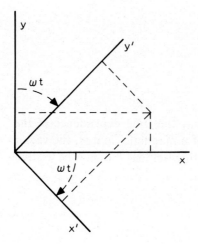

Figure 138

These three equations can be solved by introducing a new system of axes rotating with the rotating field. We introduce new axes (x'y'z'), such that z and z' coincide and x = x' cos ωt + y' sin ωt; y = −x' sin ωt + y' cos ωt. This transformation follows directly from Figure 138. An observer in the new frame (x'y'z') measures magnetizations ($M_{x'}$, $M_{y'}$, $M_{z'}$) which are related to the old ones (M_x, M_y, M_z) through

$$M_x = M_{x'} \cos \omega t + M_{y'} \sin \omega t$$

$$M_y = -M_{x'} \sin \omega t + M_{y'} \cos \omega t$$

$$M_z = M_{z'}$$

Clearly, $(dM_z/dt) = (dM_{z'}/dt)$; of the two other derivatives we only give (dM_x/dt):

$$\frac{dM_x}{dt} = \cos \omega t \, \frac{dM_{x'}}{dt} + \sin \omega t \, \frac{dM_{y'}}{dt} - \omega \sin \omega t \, M_{x'} + \omega \cos \omega t \, M_{y'}$$

Substitution, followed by elimination, leads to the 'equations of motion' of the magnetizations in the 'rotating frame'

$$\frac{d}{dt} M_{x'} + (\omega - \omega_L) M_{y'} = 0$$

$$\frac{d}{dt} M_{y'} - (\omega - \omega_L) M_{x'} = \omega_1 M_{z'}$$

$$\frac{d}{dt} M_{z'} + \omega_1 M_{y'} = 0$$

The equations are very simple for $\omega = \omega_L$, i.e., if the RF frequency coincides with the Larmor frequency,

$$\frac{d}{dt} M_{x'} = 0$$

$$\frac{d}{dt} M_{y'} - \omega_1 M_{z'} = 0$$

$$\frac{d}{dt} M_{z'} + \omega_1 M_{y'} = 0$$

From the first equation above follows: $M_{x'} = $ constant. The other two equations are satisfied by

$$M_{y'} = M \cos \omega_1 t$$

$$M_{z'} = -M \sin \omega_1 t$$

In the rotating frame the magnetization precesses about the x'-axis with frequency $\omega_1 = \gamma H_1$. Since $H_1 \ll H_0$ this precession frequency is small with respect to the Larmor frequency (Fig. 20B).

If the RF frequency and the Larmor frequency are different, the magnetization precesses about the 'effective field' (see Fig. 27C)

$$\vec{H}_{eff} = H_1 \vec{e}_x + (H_0 - \frac{\omega}{\gamma}) \vec{e}_z$$

The magnitude of H_{eff} is given by

$$H_{eff} = \sqrt{(H_0 - \frac{\omega}{\gamma})^2 + H_1^2}$$

If H_1 is strong enough ($H_0 - (\omega/\gamma/H_1) \ll 1$), then H_{eff} is practically equal to H_1 even if the resonance condition ($\omega = \omega_L$) is not met precisely: to a good approximation, the magnetization precesses about the RF field.

Appendix 6

FOURIER TRANSFORMATION OF SIGNALS MEASURED AS A FUNCTION OF TIME

It is well known that a periodic signal can be written as a sum of sine and/or cosine functions. In Figure 139 an example is given of a periodic function of one variable (which we shall identify with time),

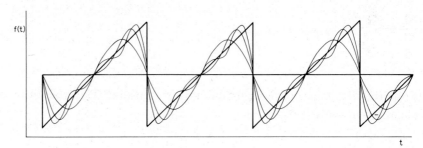

f(t)

t

Figure 139

together with its decomposition in terms of sine and cosine functions. The time-dependent function can be regarded as being made up of one basic frequency (ω) its first (2ω), second (3ω) and higher harmonics. In the example of Figure 139 the contributions of the higher harmonics decrease with the order of the harmonic.

The information contained in the time-dependent signal is equivalent to that contained in the frequency spectrum, i.e., in the 'intensities' of the contributions at the frequencies ω, 2ω, 3ω, ... The time-dependent signal is said to be Fourier-analyzed in its frequency components.

The function discussed in Figure 139 is a periodic function of time and this limitation renders the analysis relatively simple. However, most NMR signals are not periodic and one would like to enlarge the treatment of Figure 139 to aperiodic functions. A few examples will be discussed.

First, consider the time-domain spectrum of a tuning fork: it has the form of a damped oscillation (see Fig. 81). If the oscillations were not damped, the frequency spectrum would consist of a single, sharp frequency. It can be shown that the damping, i.e., the gradual decrease of the amplitude, is reflected in a finite width of the frequency spectrum: the more rapid the decay, the larger the width of the frequency spectrum, and vice versa.

Analogously, two vibrating strings with nearby frequencies give rise to a time-domain spectrum with a characteristic interference pattern (see Fig. 82). Fourier transformation leads to a frequency spectrum consisting of two lines at the two resonance frequencies of the strings. The damping introduces, as before, broadening of the two lines.

A complex, non-periodic function of time cannot be represented as a Fourier series, as in the example of Figure 139: instead, it can be represented as a Fourier integral in which the frequencies are not restricted to multiples of one basic frequency, but may vary continuously. Computer programs have been developed to handle Fourier transformations efficiently. A well-known program is denoted FFT (Fast Fourier Transform).

Mathematical representation of the Fourier integral is beyond the scope of this book; the reader is referred to books on NMR (e.g., Fourier Transform NMR Spectroscopy by Derek Shaw, Elsevier, 1984) or to mathematical texts.

References

I NMR GENERAL

Reviews, applications, environment, pulse sequences, optimization, etc.

Bakker, C. J. G. (1982) NMR characterization of tissues: Applications in radiotherapy. Symposium, Amsterdam, 27 april, 1982.

Bakker, C. J. G. and Schipper, J. (1982) Kernspinresonantie. Intermediair 50, 31–37.

Bottomley, P. A. (1982) NMR imaging techniques and applications: A review. Rev.Sci.Instrum. 53, 1319–1337.

Bottomley, P. A. (1984) NMR in medicine. Comput.Radiol. 8, 57–79.

Bradbury, E. M., Radda, G. K. and Allen, P. S. (1983) NMR techniques in medicine. Ann.Intern.Med. 98, 514–529.

Bradley, W. G. (1982) NMR tomography. Diasonics, Inc. Marketing Communications, Milpitas, CA.

Bradley, W. G., Opel, W. and Kassabian, J. P. (1984) MR installation: Siting and economic considerations. Radiology 151, 719–721.

Brady, T. J., Tyler, B. C., Goldman, M. R., Pykett, I. L., Buonanno, F. S., Kistler, J. P., Newhouse, J. H., Kinshaw, W. S. and Pohost, G. M. (1981) Tumor characterization using ^{31}P NMR spectroscopy, Symposium, Winston-Salem, NC, 1–3 October, 1981, pp. 175–180.

Budinger, T. F. (1981) Medical applications of NMR scanning. Some perspectived in relation to other techniques. Symposium, Winston-Salem, NC, 1–3 October 1981, pp. 51–63.

Budinger, T. F. (1981) NMR in vivo studies: Known thresholds for health effects. J.Comput.Assist.Tomogr. 5, 800–811.

Budinger, T. F. (1982) Dynamic transmission comp tom, emission tom, NMR methods of measuring physiologic parameters. Mayo Clin. Proc. 57, 67–78.

Bydder, G. M., Doyle, F. H., Young, I. R. and Hall, A. S. (1981) NMR initial clinical results. Symposium, Winston-Salem, NC, 1–3 October, 1981, pp. 107–113.

Bydder, G. M., Goatcher, A., Hughes, J. M. B., Orr, J. S., Pennock, J. M., Steiner, R. E. and Tripathi, A. (1982) Effect of oxygen tension on NMR spin lattice relaxation rate of blood in vivo. J.Phys. 332, 46–47.

Crooks, L. (1981) Imaging techniques. In 'Clinical Magnetic Resonance Imaging'. Ed., Margulis, A. R., Saunders, Philadelphia, pp. 25–31.

Crooks, L., Hoenninger, J., Arakawa, M., Kaufman, L., McRee, R., Watts, J. and Singer, J. H. (1980) Tomography of hydrogen with NMR. Radiology 136, 701–706.

Crooks, L., Arakawa, M., Hoenninger, J., Watts, J., McRee, R., Kaufman, L., Davis, P. L., Margulis, A. R. and De Groot, J. (1982) NMR whole-body imager operating at 3.5 KG. Radiology 143, 169–174.

172   Crooks, L., Ortendam, D. A., Kaufman, L., Hoenninger, J., Arakawa, M., Watts, J., Cannon, C. R., Brant-Zawadzki, M., David, P. L. and Margulis, A. R. (1983) Clinical efficiency of NMR. Radiology 146, 123–128.

Crooks, L., Arakawa, M., Hoenninger, J., McCarten, B., Watts. J. and Kaufman, L. (1984) MRI: effects of magnetic field strength. Radiology 151, 127–133.

Damadian, R. (1971) Tumor detection by NMR. Science 171, 1151–1153.

Davis, P. L., Crooks, L., Arakawa, M., McRee, R., Kaufman, L. and Margulis, A. R. (1981) Potential hazards in NMRI: Heating effects of changing magnetic fields and RF fields on small metallic implants. AJR 137, 857–860.

De Galan, L. (1972) Analytische Spectrometrie. Leerboek voor analysten. Heron Bibliotheek, AGON Elsevier, Amsterdam, pp. 157–175.

Dixon, R. L. and Ekstrand, K. E. (1982) The physics of proton NMR. Med. Phys. 9, 807–818.

Doyle, F. H., Gore, J. C. and Pennock, J. M. (1981) Relaxation rate enhancement observed in vivo by NMRI. J.Comput.Assist.Tomogr. 5, 295–296.

Dujovny, M., Kossovsky, N., Kossowsky, R., Diaz, F. G. and Ausman, J. I. (1983) Magnetic aneurysm clips: correlation with martensite content and implications for NMR examination. Surg.Forum 34, 525–527.

Edelstein, W. A., Hutchison, J. M. S., Smith, F. W., Mallard J., Johnson, G. and Redpath, T. H. (1981) Human whole-body NMR tomographic imaging: normal sections. Br.J.Radiol. 54, 149–151.

Epstein, F. H. (1981) NMR, a new tool in clinical medicine. N.Engl.J.Med. 28, 1360–1361.

Falke, T. H. M., Ziedses de Plantes, B. G. Jr. and Van Voorthuisen, A. E. (1984) The Netherlands initial experience with NMR imaging. Diagn.Imag.Clin.Med. 53, 43–52.

Fullerton, G. D. (1982) Basic concepts for NMR imaging. Magn.Reson.Imaging 1, 39–55.

Fullerton, G. D., Potter, J. L. and Dornbluth, N. L. (1982) NMR relaxation of protons in tissues and other macromolecular water solutions. Magn.Reson.Imaging 1, 209–226.

Fullerton, G. D., Cameron, I. L. and Ord, V. A. (1984) Frequency dependence of NMR spin-lattice relaxation of protons in biological materials. Radiology 151, 135–138.

Goldsmith, M., Koutcher, S. B. and Damadian, R. (1978) Application of the NMR malignancy-index to human gastro-intestinal tumors. Cancer 41, 183–191.

Gore, J. C. (1981) The meaning and signification of relaxation in NMR. Symposium, Winston-Salem, NC, 1–3 October, 1981, pp. 15–23.

Hanley, P. (1981) Superconducting and resistive magnets in NMR scanning. Symposium, Winston-Salem, NC, 1–3 October, 1981, pp. 41–49.

Hanley, P. (1984) Magnets for medical applications of NMR. Br.Med.Bull. 40, 125–131.

Hart, H. R., Bottomley, P. A., Edelstein, W. A., Karr, S. G., Leue, W. M., Mueller, O., Redington, R. W., Schenck, W. F., Smith, L. S. and Vatis, D. (1983) NMRI: contrast to noise ratio as a function of strength of magnetic field. AJR 141, 1195–1201.

Hilal, S. K., Einstein, S., Maudsley, A. and Silver, M. A. (1983) The merits of super-conducting magnets in NMR systems. Medica Mundi 28, 63–69.

Hoult, D. I. (1984) The sensitivity of the NMR imaging experiment. NMR in Living Systems, NATO Advanced Study Institute, Sicily.

Hounsfield, G. N. (1980) Computed medical imaging. J.Comput.Assist. Tomogr. 4, 665–674; Science 210, 22–28.

James, A. E., Price, R. R., Rollo, F. D., Partain, C. L., Patton, J. A., Erickson, J. J. and Coulam, C. M. (1982) NMR imaging, a promising technique. J.Am.Med.Assoc. 247, 1331–1334.

Katims, L. M. (1982) NMR imaging methods and current status. Med.Instrum. 16, 213–216.

Kaufman, L., Crooks, L. E. and Margulis, A. R. (1982) Nuclear Magnetic Resonance Imaging in Medicine. Igaku-Shoin, New York.

Koutcher, J. A., Goldsmith, M. and Damadian, R. (1978) A malignancy-index to discriminate normal and cancerous tissue. Cancer 41, 174–182.

Koutcher, J. A. and Tyler Burt, C. (1984) Principles of imaging by NMR. J.Nucl.Med. 25, 371–382.

Lauterbur, P. C. (1973) Image formation by induced local interactions: Examples employing NMR. Nature 242, 190–191.

Lauterbur, P. C. (1980) Progress in NMR zeugmatography imaging. Phil. Trans.R.Soc.Lond. 289, 483–487.

Laval-Jeantet, M. (1982) Imagerie par résonance magnétique nucléaire. Appl.Clin. 34, 2543–2547.

Lochner, P. R. (1983) Proton NMR tomography. Philips Techn.Rev. 41, 73–88.

Loeffler, W. and Oppelt, A. (1981) Physical principles of NMR tomography. Eur.J. Radiol. 1, 338–344.

Luiten, A. L. (1981) NMR, an introduction. Medica Mundi 26, 98–101.

Luiten, A. L., Lochner, P. R., Van Uijen, C. M. J., Van Dijk, P. and Den Boef, J. H. (1982) Clinical Results of NMR Imaging. Symposium, Amsterdam, 27 April.

Mallard, J. (1981) The Noes have it! Do they? Silvanus Thompson Memorial Lecture: February 18, 1981. Br.J.Radiol. 54, 831–849.

Mansfield, P. (1982) NMR Imaging in Biomedicine. Academic Press, London.

Menashé, P., Piwnica, A., Ingwall, J. S. and Fossel, E. T. (1981) La résonance magnétique nucléaire. Une nouvelle méthode d'évaluation des techniques de protection myocardique. Nouv. Presse Med. 10, 295–298.

New, P. J. F., Rosen, B. R., Brady, T. J., Buonanno, F. S., Kistler, J. P., Burt, C. T., Hinshaw, W. S., Newhouse, J. H., Pohost, G. M. and Taveras, J. M. (1983) Potential hazards and artifacts of ferromagnetic and nonferromagnetic surgical and dental materials and devices in NMRI. Radiology 147, 139–148.

Newton, T. H. and Gordon Potts, D. (1983) Advanced Imaging Techniques in Modern Neuroradiology, Vol. 2, Clavadel Press, San Anselmo, CA.

Ordidge, R. J., Mansfield, P. and Coupland, R. E. (1981) Rapid biomedical imaging by NMR. Br.J.Radiol. 54, 850–855.

Partain, C. L., James, A. E., Rollo, F. D. and Price, R.R. (1983) Nuclear Magnetic Resonance Imaging. W.B. Saunders Company, London.

174   Partain, C. L. et al. (1984) Nuclear Magnetic Resonance and Correlative Imaging Modalities. The Society of Nuclear Medicine, New York.

Pavlicek, W., Geisinger, M., Castle, L., Borkowsky, G.P., Meany, T. F., Bream, B. L. and Gallagher, J. H. (1983), The effects of NMR on patients with cardiac pacemakers. Radiology 147, 149–153.

Prasad, N., Buskong, S. C., Thornby, J. I., Bryan, R. N., Hazelwood, C. F. and Harrell, J. E. (1984) Effect of nuclear magnetic resonance on chromosomes of mouse bone marrow cells. Magn.Reson.Imaging 2, 37–39.

Pykett, I. L. (1980) NMR imaging, a new technique for the study of intact biological systems. Eur.Spectroscopy News 33, 19–22.

Pykett, I. L. (1982) NMR imaging in medicine. Sci.Am. 5, 54–64.

Reid, A., Smith, F. W. and Hutchison, J. M. S. (1982) NMR imaging and its safety implications: follow-up of 181 patients. Br.J.Radiol. 55, 784–786.

Roth, K. (1984) NMR-tomographie und NMR-spektroskopie in der Medizin. Eine Einführing. Springer Verlag, Berlin.

Runge, V. M., Clanton, J. A., Partain, C. L. and James, A. E. (1984) Respiratory gating in MRI at 0.5 T. Radiology 151, 521–523.

Saunders, R. D. (1982) Biology effects of NMR clinical imaging. Appl.Radiol. 11, 43.

Schultz, C. L., Alfidi, R. J., Nelson, A. D., Kopiwoda, S. Y. and Clampitt, M. E. (1984) The effect of motion on two-dimensional Fourier transformation magnetic resonance images. Radiology 152, 117–121.

Scott, A. (1981) NMR spot the atom, watch the cell. New Sci. 92, 440–443.

Scott, A. (1982) NMR, a technique whose time has come. New Sci. 94, 213.

Sepponen, R. E., Sipponen, J. T. and Tanttu, J. I. (1984) A method for chemical shift imaging: demonstration of bone marrow involvement with proton chemical shift imaging. J.Comput.Assist.Tomogr. 8, 585–587.

Shulman, R. D. (1983) NMR spectroscopy of living cells. Sci.Am. 248, 86–93.

Smith, F. W. (1981) Clinical application of NMR tomographic imaging. Symposium, Winston-Salem, NC, 1–3 October, 1981, pp. 125–132.

Smith, F. W. (1982) Safety of NMR imaging. Lancet I, 974.

Visser, R. (1972) Structuuropheldering van Organische Verbindingen met Behulp van Spectrometrische Methoden. Heron Bibliotheek, AGON Elsevier, Amsterdam, pp. 92–126.

Wehrli, F. W., McFall, J. R., Glover, G. H. and Grigsby, N. (1984) The dependence of nuclear magnetic resonance (NMR) image contrast on intrinsic and pulse sequence; timing parameters. Magn.Reson.Imaging 2, 3–16.

Wolff, S., Crooks, L. E., Brown, P., Howard, R. and Painter, R. B. (1980) Tests for DNA and chromosomal damage induced by NMRI. Radiology 136, 707–710.

Young, S. W. (1984) Nuclear Magnetic Resonance; Basic Principles. Raven Press, New York.

Zuiderweg, E. (1979) Een fysische methode voor chemisch en biochemisch structuuronderzoek. Natuur en Techniek 47, 50–67.

Brasch, R. C. (1983) Work in progress: methods of contrast enhancement for NMRI and potential applications. Radiology 147, 781–788.

Brown, M. A. and Johnson, G. A. (1984) Transition metal-chelate complexes as relaxation modifices in NMR. Med.Phys. 11, 67–72.

Bydder, G. M., Goatcher, A., Hughes, J. M. B., Orr, J. S., Pennock, J. M., Steiner, R. E. and Tripathi, A. (1982) Effect of oxygen tension on NMR spin lattice relaxation rate of blood in vivo. J.Phys. 332, 46–47.

Carr, D. H., Brown, J., Bydder, G. M., Steiner, R. E., Weinman, H. J., Speck, U., Hall, A. S. and Young, I. R. (1984) Gadolinium-DTPA a a contrast agent in MRI. AJR 143, 215–244.

Carr, D. H., Bydder, G. M. and Brown, J. (1984) Intravenous chelated gadolinium as a contrast agent in NMR; imaging of cerebral tumours. Lancet I, 484–486.

Grossman, R. I., Wolf, G., Biery, D., McGrath, J., Kundel, H., Aronchick, J., Zimmerman, A., Goldberg, H. I. and Bilaniuk, L. T. (1984) Gadolinium enhanced NMR images of experimental brain abscess. J.Comput.Assist.Tomogr. 8, 204–207.

Koutcher, J. A., Tyler Burt, C., Lauffer, R. B. and Brady, T. J. (1984) Contrast agent and spectroscopic probes in NMR. J.Nucl.Med. 25, 506–513.

Runge, V. M., Foster, M. A., Clanton, J. A., Jones, M. M., Lukehart, C. M., Hutchison, J. M. S., Mallard, J. R., Smith, F. W., Partain, C. L. and James, A. E. (1984) Contrast enhancement of magnetic resonance images by chromium EFTA: an experimental study. Radiology 152, 123–126.

II   CLINICAL APPLICATIONS OF NMR

General

Alfidi, R. J., Haaga, J. R., El Yousef, S. J., Bryen, P. J., Fletcher, B. D., Li Puma, J. P., Morrison, S. C., Kaufman, B., Richey, J. B., Hinshaw, W. S., Kramer, D. M., Yeung, H. N., Coker, A. M., Butler, H. E., Arment, A. E. and Lieberman, J. M. (1982) Preliminary experimental results in humans and animals with a superconducting, whole-body NMR scanner. Radiology 143, 175–181.

Hansen, G., Crooks, L. E., Davis, P., De Groot, J., Herfkens, R., Margulis, A. R., Gooding, C., Kaufman, L., Hoeninger, J., Arakawa, M., McRee, R. and Watts, J. (1980) In vivo imaging of the rat anatomy with NMR. Radiology 136, 695–700.

Hinshaw, W. S., Andrew, E. R., Bottomley, P. P., Holland, G. N. and Moore, W. S. (1978) Display of cross sectional anatomy by NMR. Br.J.Radiol. 51, 273–280.

Pollet, J. E., Smith, F. W., Mallard, J. R., Ah-See, A. K. and Reid, A. (1981) Whole-body NMRI: the first report of its use in surgical practice. Br.J.Surg. 68, 493–494.

Young, I. R., Bailes, D. R., Burl, M., Collins, A. G., Smith, D. T., McDonnell, M. J., Orr, J. S., Banks, L. M., Bydder, G. M., Greenspan, R. H. and Steiner, R. E. (1982) Initial clinical evaluation of a whole-body NMR tomograph. J.Comput.Assist.Tomogr. 6, 1–18.

Brain

Anderson, M. (1982) NMR imaging and neurology. Br.Med.J. 284, 1359–1360.

Bottomley, P.A., Foster, T.H. and Leue, W.M. (1984) Chemical imaging of the brain by NMR. Lancet I, 1120.

Brant-Zawadzki, M., Davis, P. L., Crooks, L. E., Mills, C. M., Norman, D., Newton, T. H., Sheldon, D. and Kaufman, L. (1983) NMR demonstration of cerebral abnormalities: comparison with CT. AJR 140, 847–854.

Brant-Zawadzki, M., Norman, D., Newton, T. H., Kelly, W. M., Kjos, B., Mills, C. M., Dillon, W., Sobel, D. and Crooks, L. E. (1984) Magnetic resonance of the brain: the optimal screening technique. Radiology 152, 71–77.

Bydder, G. M. (1983) Brain imaging by NMR. Practitioner 227, 497–501.

Bydder, G. M. (1984) NMR imaging of the brain. Br.Med.Bull. 40, 170–175.

Bydder, G. M. and Steiner, R. E. (1982) NMR imaging of the brain. Neuroradiology 23, 231–240.

Bydder, G. M., Steiner, R. E., Young, I. R., Hall, A. S., Thomas, D. J., Marshall, J., Pallis, C. A. and Legg, N. J. (1982) Clinical NMR imaging of the brain: 140 cases. AJNR 3, 459–480.

Cady, E. B., Costello, A. M. De L., Dawson, J. M., Delpy, D. T., Hope, P. I., Reynolds, E. O. R., Tofts, P. S. and Wilkie, D. R. (1983) Noninvasive investigation of cerebral metabolism in newborn infants by P-NMR spectroscopy. Lancet 1, 1059–1062.

Doyle, F. H., Gore, J. C., Pennock, J. M., Bydder, G. M., Orr, J. S. and Steiner, R. E. (1981) Imaging of the brain by NMR. Lancet 11, 53–57.

Erkinjuntti, T., Sipponen, J. T., Iivanainen, M., Ketonen, L., Sulkava, R. and Sepponen, R. E. (1984) Cerebral NMR and CT imaging in dementia. J.Comput.Assist.Tomogr. 8, 614–618.

Hawkes, R. C., Holland, G. N., Moore, W. S. and Worthington, B. S. (1980) NMR tomography of the brain: a preliminary clinical assessment with demonstration of pathology. J.Comput.Assist.Tomogr. 4, 577–586.

Hawkes, R. C., Holland, G. N., Moore, W. S., Corston, R., Kean, D. M. and Worthington, B. S. (1983) Craniovertebral junction pathology; assessment by NMR. AJNR 4, 232–233.

Holland, G. N., Hawkes, R. C. and Moore, W. S. (1980) NMR tomography of the brain: coronal and sagittal sections. J.Comput.Assist.Tomogr. 4, 429–433.

Holland, G. N., Moore, W. S. and Hawkes, R. C. (1980) NMR tomography of the brain. J.Comput.Assist.Tomogr. 4, 1–3.

Holland, G. N., Moore, W. S. and Hawkes, R. C. (1980) NMR neuroradiography. Br.J.Radiol. 53, 253–255.

Huk, H., Heindel, W., Deimling, M. and Stetter, E. (1983) NMR tomography of the central nervous system: comparison of two imaging sequences. J.Comput.Assist.Tomogr. 7, 468–475.

Johnson, M. A. and Bydder, G. M. (1984) NMR imaging of the brain in children. Br.Med.Bull. 40, 175–179.

Johnson, M. A., Pennock, J. M., Bydder, G. M., Steiner, R. E., Thomas, D. J., Hayward, R., Bryant, D. R. T., Dayne, J. A., Levene, M. I., Whitelaw, A., Dubowitz, L. M. S. and Dubowitz, V. (1983) Clinical NMR imaging of the brain in children: normal and neurologic disease. AJNR 4, 1013–1026.

Levene, M. I., Whitelaw, A., Dubowitz, V., Bydder, G. M., Steiner, R. E., Randell, C. P. and Young, I. R. (1982) NMR imaging of the brain in children. Br.Med.J. 285, 774–776.

Lukes, S. A., Aminoff, M. J., Crooks, L., Kaufman, L., Mills, C. and Newton, T. H. (1983) NMR imaging in movement disorders. Ann.Neurol. 13, 592–601.

Mills, C. M., Crooks, L. E., Kaufman, L. and Brant-Zawadzki, M. (1984) Cerebral abnormalities: use of calculated T_1 and T_2 magnetic resonance images for diagnosis. Radiology 150, 87–94.

Simmonds, D., Banks, L. M., Steiner, R. E. and Young, I. R. (1983) NMR anatomy of the brain using IR sequences. Neuroradiology 25, 113–118.

Stark, D. D., Moss, A. A., Gamsu, G., Clark, O. H., Gooding, G. A. W. and Webb, W. R. (1984) MRI of the neck; normal anatomy and pathologic findings. Radiology 150, 447–461.

Tishler, J. M. A. and Partain, C. L. (1984) NMR of the CNS. Ala.J.Med.Sci. 21, 190–103.

Young, I. R., Burl, M., Clarke, G. J., Hall, A. S., Pasmore, T., Collins, A. G., Smith, D. T., Orr, J. S., Bydder, G. M., Doyle, F. H., Greenspan, R. H. and Steiner, R. E. (1981) Magnetic resonance properties of hydrogen. Imaging the posterior fossa. AJR 137, 895–901.

Younkin, D. P., Leonard, J. C., Delivori, M., Subraman, H., and Chance, B. (1983) Unique features of human newborn cortical metabolism measured with ^{31}P-NMR. Ann.Neurol. 14, 355–355.

Zimmerman, R. A., Bilaniuk, L. T., Goldberg, H. I., Grossman, R. I., Levine, R. S., Lynch, R., Edelstein, W., Bottomley, P. and Redington, R. (1984) Cerebral imaging. AJNR 5, 1–7.

Vascular disorders

Asato, R., Handa, H., Hashi, T., Hatta, J., Komoike, M. and Yanaki, T. (1983) Chronological sequences and bloodbrain barrier permeability changes in local injury as assessed by NMR images of sliced rat brain. Stroke 14, 191–197.

Bryan, R. N., Willcott, M. R., Schneiders, N. J., Ford, J. J. and Derman, H. S. (1983) NMR evaluation of stroke. Radiology 149, 189–192.

Bryan, R. N., Willcott, M. R., Schneiders, N. J. and Rose, J. E. (1983) NMR evaluation of stroke in the rat. AJNR 4, 242–244.

Buonanno, F. S., Pykett, I. L., Kistler, J. P., Vielma, J., Brady, T. J., Hinshaw, W. S., Goldman, M. R., Newhouse, J. H. and Pohost, G. M. (1982) Cranial anatomy and detection of ischemic stroke in the cat by NMR imaging. Radiology 143, 187–193.

Crooks, L., Mills, C. M., Davis, P. L., Brant-Zawadzki, M., Hoenninger, J., Arakawa, M., Watts, G. and Kaufman, L. (1982) Visualization of cerebral and vascular abnormalities by NMR imaging. The effect of imaging parameters on contrast. Radiology 144, 843–852.

178 DeLaPaz, R. L., New, P. F. J., Buonanno, F. J., Kistler, J. P., Oot, R. F., Rosen, B. R., Traveras, J. M. and Brady, T. J. (1984) NMR imaging of intracranial hemorrhage. J.Comput.Assist.Tomogr. 8, 599–607.

Delpy, D. T., Gordon, R. E., Hope, P. L., Parker, D., Reynolds, E. O. R., Shaw, D. and Whitehead, H. D. (1982) Non invasive investigation of cerebral ischaemia by phosphor NMR. Pediatrics 70, 310–313.

Hilal, S. K., Maudsley, A. A., Simon, H. E., Perman, W. H., Bonn, J., Mawad, M. E., Silver, A. J., Ganti, S. R., Sane, D. and Chieu, I. C. (1983) In vivo NMR imaging of tissue sodium in the intact cat before and after acute cerebral stroke. AJNR 4, 245–249.

Kistler, J. P., Buonanno, F. S., DeWitt, L. D., Davies, K. R., Brady, T. J. and Fisher, C. M. (1984) Vertebral-basilair posterior cerebral territory stroke. Delineation by NMR I. Stroke 15, 417–426.

Levy, R. M., Mano, I., Brito, A. and Hosobuchi, Y. (1983) NMR imaging of acute experimental cerebral ischemia: time course and pharmacological manipulat ons. AJNR 4, 238–241.

Mano, I., Levy, R. M., Crooks, L. E. and Hosobuchi, Y. (1983) NMRI of acute experimental cerebral ischemia. Invest.Radiol. 18, 345–351.

Moon, K. L., Brant-Zawadzki, M., Pitts, L. H. and Mills, C. M. (1984) NMR of CT isodense subdural hematomas. AJNR 5, 319–323.

Pykett, I. L., Buonanno, F. S., Brady, T. J. and Kistler, J. P. (1983) True 2-D NMR neuroimaging in ischemic stroke correlation of NMR X-ray CT and pathology. Stroke 14, 173–177.

Sipponen, J. T., Kaste, M., Sepponen, R. E., Kuurne, T., Suoranta, H. and Sivula, N. J. (1983) NMR imaging in reversible cerebral ischaemia. Lancet I, 294–295.

Sipponen, J. T., Kaste, M., Ketonen, L., Sepponen, R. E., Katevuo, K. and Sivula, A. (1983) Serial NMR imaging in patients with cerebral infarction. J.Comput.Assist.Tomogr. 7, 585–589.

Sipponen, J. T., Sepponen, R. E. and Sivula, A. (1983) NMR imaging of intra-cerebral hemorrhage in the acute and resolving phases. J.Comput.Assist.Tomogr. 7, 954–959.

Sipponen, J. T., Sepponen, R. E. and Sivula, A. (1984) Chronic subdural hematoma: demonstration by magnetic resonance. Radiology 150, 79–85.

Spetzler, R. F., Zabramski, J. M., Kaufman, B. and Yeung, H. N. (1983) Acute NMR changes during MCA occlusion: a preliminary study. Stroke 14, 185–191.

Worthington, B. S., Kean, D. M., Hawkes, R. C., Holland, G. N., Moore, W. S. and Corston, R. (1983) NMRI in the recognition of giant intracranial aneurysms. AJNR 4, 835–836.

Tumours

Aaron, J., New, P. F. J., Strand, R., Beaulieu, P., Elunden, K. and Brady, T. J. (1984) NMR imaging in temporal lobe epilepsy due to gliomas. J.Comput.Assist.Tomogr. 8, 608–613.

Araki, T., Inouye, T., Suzuki, H., Mochida, T. and Iio, M. (1984) Magnetic resonance imaging of brain tumors: measurement of T_1. Radiology 150, 95–98.

Brady, T. J., Buonanno, F. S., Pykett, I. L., New, P. F. J., Davis, K. R., Pohost, G. M. and Kistler, J. P. (1983) Preliminary clinical results of proton (^{1}H) imaging of cranial neoplasms: in vivo measurements of T_1 and mobile proton density. AJNR 4, 225–228.

Brant-Zawadzki, M., Badami, J. P., Mills, C. M., Norman, D. and Newton, T. H. (1984) Primary intracranial tumor imaging: a comparison of MR and CT. Radiology 150, 435–550.

Buonanno, F. S., Pykett, I. L., Brady, T. J., Black, P., New, P. F. J., Richardson, E. P., Hinshaw, W. S., Goldman, M., Pohost, G. and Kistler, J. P. (1982) Clinical relevance of two different NMR approaches to imaging of a lowgrade astrocytoma. J.Comput.Assist.Tomogr. 6, 529–535.

Hawkes, R. C., Holland, G. N., Moore, W. S., Gorston, R., Kean, D. M. and Worthington, B. S. (1983) The application of NMR imaging to the evaluation of pituitary and juxtasellar tumors. AJNR 4, 221–222.

McGinnis, B. D., Brady, T. J., New, P. F. J., Buonanno, F. S., Pykett, I. L., DeLaPaz, R. L., Kistler, J. P. and Taveras, J. M. (1983) NMR imaging of tumors in the posterior fossa. J.Comput.Assist.Tomogr. 7, 575–584.

Oot, R., New, P. F. J., Buonanno, F. S., Pykett, I. L., Kistler, P., DeLaPaz, R., Davis, K. R., Taveras, J. M. and Brady, T. J. (1984) MR imaging of pituitary adenomas using a prototype resistive magnet. AJNR 5, 131–137.

Packer, R. J., Zimmerman, R. A., Bilaniuk, L. B., Sutton, L. N., Rosensto, J. G., Bruce, D. A., Schut, L., Reddington, R. W. and Edelstein, W. (1983) NMR of childhood brain tumors. Ann.Neurol. 14, 371.

Randell, C. P., Collius, A. G., Young, I. R., Haywood, R., Thomas, D. J., McDonnell, M. J., Orr, J. S., Bydder, G. M. and Steiner, R. E. (1983) NMR imaging of posterior fossa tumors. AJNR 4, 1027–1034.

Von Einsiedel, H. G. and Löffler, W. (1982) NMR imaging of a brain tumor unrevealed by CT. Eur.J.Radiol. 2, 226–235.

Von Stober, T., Huber, G. and Huk, W. (1983) Kernspintomogramm eines im CCT nur unzureichend dargestellten Germinoms. ROEFO 139, 648–650.

Weinstein, M. A., Modic, M. T., Pavlicek, W. and Keyser, C. K. (1984) NMR for the examination of brain tumors. Semin.Roetgenol. 19, 139–147.

Young, I. R., Bydder, G. M., Hall, A. S., Steiner, R. E., Worthington, B. S., Hawkes, R. C., Holland, G. N. and Moore, W. S. (1983) The role of NMR imaging in the diagnosis and management of acoustic neuroma. AJNR 4, 223–224.

Disorders of myelinization

Bradley, W. G. (1984) Patchy periventricular white matter lesions in the elderly: a common observation during NMRI. Noninvasive Imaging 1, 35–42.

Lukes, S. A., Crooks, L. E., Aminoff, M. J., Kaufman, L., Panitch, H. S., Mills, C. and Norman, D. (1983) NMR imaging in multiple sclerosis. Ann.Neurol. 13, 592–601.

Mastaglia, F. L. and Cala, L. A. (1982) NMR and CT in multiple sclerosis. Lancet I, 850.

Young, I. R., Hall, A. S., Pallis, C. A., Legg, N. J., Bydder, G. M. and Steiner, R. E. (1981) NMR imaging of the brain in multiple sclerosis. Lancet II, 1063–1066.

180   Young, I. R., Randell, C. P., Kaplan, P. W., James, A., Bydder, G. M. and Steiner, R. E. (1983) NMR imaging in white matter disease of the brain using spin-echo sequences. J.Comput.Assist.Tomogr. 7, 290–294.

Miscellaneous

Brant-Zawadzki, M., Enzmann, D. R., Placone, R. C., Sheldon, P., Britt, R. H., Brasch, R. C. and Crooks, L. (1983) NMR imaging of experimental brain abscess: comparison with CT. AJNR 4, 250–253.

Brant-Zawadzki, M., Bartkowski, H. M., Ortendahl, D. A., Pitts, L. H., Hylton, N. M., Nishimura, M. C. and Crooks, L. E. (1984) NMR in experimental cerebral edema: Value of T_1 and T_2 calculations. AJNR 5, 125–129.

Daniels, D. L., Herfkins, R., Gager, W. E., Meyer, G. A., Koehler, P. R., Williams, A. L. and Haughton, V. M. (1984) Radiology 152, 79–83.

Daniels, D. L., Herfkins, R., Koehler, P. R., Millen, S. J., Shaffer, K. A., Williams, A. L. and Haughton, V. M. (1984) MRI of the internal auditory canal. Radiology 151, 105–108.

DeLaPaz, R. L., Brady, T. J., Buonanno, F. S., New, P. F. J., Kistler, J. P., McGinnis, B. D., Pykett, I. L. and Taveras, J. M. (1983) NMR imaging of Arnold-Chiari type I malformation with hydromyelie. J.Comput.Assist.Tomogr. 7, 126–129.

DeWitt, L. D., Buonanno, F. S., Kistler, J. P., Zeffiro, T., DeLaPaz, R. L., Brady, T. J., Rosen, B. R. and Pykett, I. L. (1984) Central Pontine Myelinolysis – Demonstration by NMR. Neurology 34, 570–576.

Go, K. G., Piers, A., Van Woerden, H. and Gerlam, H. (1982) NMR case study: Arachnoid cyst diagnosis. Medica Mundi 27, 41–42.

Greiner, J. V., Kopp, S. J. and Glonek, T. (1984) Nondestructive metabolic analysis of a cornea with the use of P-NMR. Arch.Opthalmol. 102, 770–771.

Grossman, R. I., Wolf, G., Bierry, D., McGrath, J., Kundel, H., Aronchick, J., Zimmerman, R. A., Goldberg, H. I. and Bilaniuk, L. T. (1984) Gadolinium enhanced NMR images of experimental brain abscess. J.Comput.Assist.Tomogr. 8, 204–207.

Han, J. S., Kaufman, B., Alfidi, R. L., Yeung, H. N., Benson, J. E., Haaga, J. R., El Yousef, S. J., Clampitt, M. E., Bonstelle, C. T. and Huss, R. (1984) Head trauma evaluated by magnetic resonance and CT: a comparison. Radiology 150, 71–77.

Hawkes, R. C., Holland, G. N., Moore, W. S., Rizk, S., Worthington, B. S. and Kean, D. M. (1983) NMRI in the evaluation of orbital tumors. AJNR 4, 254–256.

Jolesz, F. A., Polak, J. F., Ruenzel, P. W. and Adams, D. F. (1984) Wallerian degeneration demonstrated by magnetic resonance: spectroscopic measurements on peripheral nerve. Radiology 152, 85–87.

Lukes, S. A., Norman, D. and Mills, C. (1983) Acute disseminated encephalomyelitis CT and NMR findings. J.Comput.Assist.Tomogr. 7, 182.

Moseley, I., Brant-Zawadzki, M. and Mills, C. (1983) NMR of the orbit. Br.J.Opthalmol. 67, 333–342.

Naruse, S., Yoshiharu, H., Tanaka, C., Hirakawa, K., Nishikawa, H. and Yoshizaki, K. (1982) Proton NMR studies on brain edema. J.Neurosurg. 56, 747–752.

Vermess, M., Bernstein, R. M., Bydder, G. M., Steiner, R. E., Young, I. R., and Hughes, G. R. V. (1983) NMR imaging of the brain in systemic lupus erythematosus. J.Comput.Assist.Tomogr. 7, 461–467.

Chafetz, N. I., Genant, H. K., Moon, K. L., Helms, C. A. and Morris, J. H. (1984) Recognition of lumbar disk herniation with NMR. AJNR 5, 23–26.

Han, J. S., Kaufman, B., El Yousef, S. J., Benson, J. E., Bonstelle, C. T., Alfidi, R. J., Haaga, R. J. , Yeung, H. and Russ, R. G. (1983) NMR imaging of the spine. AJNR 4, 1151–1159.

Jolesz, F. A., Polak, J. F., Ruenzel, P. W. and Adams, D. F. (1984) Wallerian degeneration demonstrated by magnetic resonance: spectroscopic measurements on peripheral nerve. Radiology 152, 85–87.

Modic, M. T. and Weinstein, M. A. (1984) NMR of the spine. Br.Med.Bull. 40, 183–187.

Modic, M. T., Weinstein, M. A., Pavlicek, W., Starnes, D. L., Duchesneau, P. M., Boumphrey, F. and Harcey, R. (1983) NMR imaging of the spine. Radiology 148, 757–762.

Modic, M. T., Pavlicek, W., Weinstein, M. A., Boumphrey, F., Ngo, F., Hardy, R. and Duchesneau, P. M. (1984) Magnetic resonance imaging in intervertebral disk disease. Radiology 152, 103–111.

Modic, M. T., Weinstein, M. A., Pavlicek, W., Boumphrey, F., Starnes, D. L. and Duchesneau, P. M. (1984) MRI of the cervical spine. AJNR 5, 15–22.

Norman, D., Mills, C. M., Brant-Zawadzki, M., Yeates, A., Crooks, L. E. and Kaufman, L. (1984) MRI of the spinal cord and canal. AJNR 5, 9–14.

Smith, F. W., Runge, V., Permezel, M. and Smith, C. C. (1984) Nuclear magnetic resonance (NMR) imaging in the diagnosis of spinal osteomyelitis. Magn.Reson.Imaging. 2, 53–56.

Yeates, A., Brant-Zawadzki, M., Norman, D., Kaufman, L., Crooks, L. E. and Newton, T. H. (1983) NMR imaging of syringomyelia. AJNR 4, 234–237.

Myopathy
Arnold, D. L., Bore, P. J., Radda, G. K., Styles, P. and Taylor, D. J. (1984) Excessive intracellular acidosis skeletal muscle on exercise in a patient with a postviral exhaustion/fatigue syndrome. Lancet I, 1367–1369.

Edwards, R. H. T., Joan Dawson, M., Wilkie, D. R., Gordon. R. E. and Shaw, D. (1982) Clinical use of NMR in the investigation of myopathy. Lancet I, 725–730.

Gadian, D., Radda, G., Ross, B., Hockaday, J., Bore, P., Taylor, D. J. and Styles, P. (1981) Examination of a myopathy by P-31 NMR. Lancet II, 774–775.

Herfkens, R. J., Sievers, R., Kaufman, L., Sheldon, P. E., Ortendahl, D. A., Lipton, M. J., Crooks, L. E. and Higgins, C. B. (1983) NMR imaging of the infarcted muscle; a rat model. Radiology 147, 761–764.

Misra, L. K., Kasturi, S. R., Kunau, S. K., Harati, Y., Mazlewood, C. T. and Luthra, M. G. (1982) Evaluation of muscle degeneration in inherited muscular dystrophy by nuclear magnetic resonance techniques. Magn.Reson. Imaging 1, 75–79.

Misra, L. K., Luthra, M. G., Amtey, S. R., Elizondo-Riojas, G., Swezey, S. H. and Todd, L. E. (1984) Enhanced T_1 differentiation between normal and dystrophic muscles. Magn.Reson.Imaging 2, 33–35.

Moon, K. L., Genant, H. K., Helms, C. A., Chafetz, N. I., Crooks, L. E. and Kaufman, L. (1983) Musculo skeletal applications of NMR. Radiology 147, 161–181.

182 Newman, R. J., Bore, P. J., Chan, L., Gadian, D. G., Styles, P., Taylor, D. and Radda, G. K. (1982) NMR studies of forearm muscle in Duchenne dystrophy. Br.Med.J. 284, 1072–1074.

Ross, B. D., Radda, G. K., Gadian, D. G., Rocker, G., Esiri, M. and Falconer-Smith, J. (1981) Examination of a case of suspected McArdle's syndrome by P-31 NMR. New.Engl.J.Med. 304, 1338–1342.

Tayler, R. G., Bogusky, R. T. and Lieberma, J. S. (1984) NMR spectroscopy for diagnosis of McArdle disease. West.J.Med. 140, 607.

Cardiology

Heart and great vessels

Axel, L., Herman, G. T., Udupa, J. K., Bottomley, P. A. and Edelstein, W. A. (1983) 3-Dimensional display of NMR cardiovascular images. J.Comput.Assist.Tomogr. 7, 172–174.

Crooks, L., Sheldon, P., Kaufman, L., Rowan, W. and Miller, T. (1982) Quantification of obstructions in vessels by NMR. IEEE Trans.Nucl.Sci. 29, 1181–1185.

De Layre, J. L., Ingwall, J. S., Malloy, C. and Fossel, E. T. (1981) Gated sodium-23 NMR images of an isolated perfused working rat heart. Science 212, 935–936.

Doyle, M., Rzedzian, R. and Mansfield, P. (1983) Dynamic NMR cardiac imaging in a piglet. Br.J.Radiol. 56, 925–930.

Dujovny, M., Kossovsky, N., Kossowsky, R., Diaz, F. G. and Ausman, J. I. (1983) Magnetic aneurysm clips: correlation with martensite content and implications for NMR examination. Surg.Forum 34, 525–527.

Fletcher, B. G., Jacobstein, M. D., Nelson, A. D., Riemenschneider, T. A. and Alfidi, R. J. (1984) Gated magnetic resonance imaging of congenital cardiac malformations. Radiology 150, 137–140.

Go, R. T., McIntyre, W. J., Yeung, H. N., Kramer, D. M., Geisinger, M., Chilcote, W., George, C., O'Donnell, J. K., Moodie, D. S. and Meany, T. J. (1984) Volume and planar gated cardiac magnetic resonance imaging: a correlative study of normal anatomy with thallium-201 spect and cadaver sections. Radiology 150, 129–135.

Hawkes, R. C., Holland, G. N., Moore, W. S., Roebuck, E. J. and Worthington, B. S. (1981) NMR tomography of the normal heart and abdomen. J.Comput.Assist.Tomogr. 5, 605–618.

Herfkens, R. J., Higgins, C. B., Hricak, H., Lipton, M. J., Crooks, L. E., Lanzer, P., Botvinick, E., Brundage, B., Sheldon, P. E. and Kaufman, L. (1983) NMR imaging of the cardiovascular system: normal and pathologic findings. Radiology 147, 749–759.

Herfkens, R. J., Higgins, C. B., Hricak, H., Lipton, M. J., Crooks, L. E., Sheldon, P. E. and Kaufman, L. (1983) NMRI of atherosclerotic disease. Radiology 148, 161–166.

Jacobstein, M. D., Fletcher, B. D., Nelson, A. D., Goldstein, S., Alfidi, R. J. and Riemenschneider, T. A. (1984) ECG gated MRI: Appearance of the congenitally malformed heart. Am.Heart J. 107, 1014–1020.

Jacobus, W. E., Taylor, G. J., Hollis, D. P. and Nunnally, R. L. (1977) Phosphorus NMR of perfused working rat hearts. Nature 265, 756–758.

Kaufman, L., Crooks, L. E., Sheldon, P. E., Rowan, W. and Miller, T. (1982) Evaluation of NMR imaging for detection and quantification of obstruction in vessels. Invest.Radiol. 17, 554–560.

Kaufman, L., Crooks, L., Sheldon, P., Hricak, H., Herfkens, R. and Bank, W. (1983) The potential impact of NMR imaging on cardiovascular diagnosis. Circulation 67, 251–257.

Lanzer, P., Botvinick, E. H., Schiller, N. B., Crooks, L. E., Arakawa, M., Kaufman, L., Davis, P. L., Herfkens, R., Lipton, M. G. and Higgins, C. B. (1984) Cardiac imaging using gated magnetic resonance. Radiology 150, 121–127.

Lieberman, J. M., Alfidi, R. J., Nelson, A. D., Botti, R. E., Moir, T. W., Haaga, J. R., Kopiwoda, S., Miraldi, F. O., Cohen, A. M., Butler, H. E., Nara, A. and Hellerstein, H. K. (1984) Gated magnetic resonance imaging of the normal and diseased heart. Radiology 152, 465–470.

Pernot, A. C., Ingwall, J. S., Menasche, P., Grousset, C., Bercot, M., Piwnica, A. and Fossel, E. T. (1983) Evaluation of high-energy metabolism during cardioplegic arrest and reperfusion – a phosphorus 31 NMR study. Circulation 67, 1296–1303.

Pohost, G. M. and Ratner, A. V. (1984) NMR potential applications in clinical cardiology. J.Am.Med.Assoc. 251, 1304–1309.

Radda, G. K. (1983) Potential and limitations of NMR for the cardiologist. Br.Heart J. 50, 197–201.

Stark, D. D., Higgins, C. B., Lanzer, P., Lipton, M. J., Schiller, N., Crooks, L. E., Botvinick, E. B. and Kaufman, L. (1984) MRI of the pericardium: Normal and pathologic findings. Radiology 150, 469–474.

Steiner, R. E. (1984) NMR imaging of the heart and mediastinum. Br.Med.Bull. 40, 191–194.

Steiner, R. E., Bydder, G. M., Selwyn, A., Deanfield, J., Longmore, D. B., Klipstein, R. H. and Firmin, D. (1983) NMR imaging of the heart. Br.Heart J. 50, 202–208.

Van Dijk, P. (1984) ECG triggered NMRI of the heart. Diagn.Imaging Clin.Med. 53, 29–37.

Van Dijk, P. (1984) Direct cardiac NMRI of heart wall and blood flow velocity. J.Comput.Assist.Tomogr. 18, 429–437.

Walpoth, B. H. (1983) Assessment of myocardial compliance and energy reserve (NMR) after hypothermic storage for 24 hours. Surg.Forum 34, 244–247.

Infarct

Brady, T. J., Goldman, M. R., Pykett, I. L., Buonanno, F. S., Kistler, J. P., Newhouse, J. H., Burt, C. T., Hinshaw, W. S. and Pohost, G. M. (1982) Proton NMRI of regionally ischemic canine hearts: effects of paramagnetic proton signal enhancement. Radiology 144, 343–347.

Buonanno, F. S., Pykett, I. L., Brady, T. J., Vielma, J., Burt, C. T., Goldman, M. R., Hinshaw, W. S., Pohost, G. M. and Kistler, J. P. (1983) Proton NMR imaging in experimental ischemic infarction. Stroke 14, 178–184.

Frank, J. A., Feiler, M. A., House, W. V., Lauterbur, P. C. and Jacobson, M. J. (1976) Measurement of proton NMR longitudinal relaxation time and water content in infarcted canine myocardium and induced pulmonary injury. Clin.Res. 24, 217A.

Goldman, M. R., Fossel, E. T., Ingwall, J. S. and Pohost, G. M. (1981) Use of 19-F NMR for evaluation of ischemic and infarcted myocardium. J.Comput.Assist.Tomogr. 5, 304.

184   Goldman, M. R., Brady, T. J., Pykett, I. L., Burt, C. T., Buonanno, F. S., Kistler, J. P., Newhouse, J. H., Hinshaw, W. S. and Pohost, G. M. (1982) Quantification of experimental myocardial infarction using NMR imaging and paramagnetic ion contrast enhancement in excised canine hearts. Circulation 66, 1012–1016.

Herfkens, R. J., Sievers, R., Kaufman, L., Sheldon, P. E., Ortendahl, D. A., Lipton, M. J., Crooks, L. E. and Higgins, C. B. (1983) NMR imaging of the infarcted muscle; a rat model. Radiology 147, 761–764.

Higgins, C. B., Herfkens, R., Lipton, M. J., Sievers, R., Sheldon, P., Kaufman, L. and Crooks, L.E. (1983) NMRI of acute myocardial infarction in dogs: alteration in magnetic relaxation times. Am.J.Cardiol. 54, 184–188.

Higgins, C. B., Lanzer, P., Stark, D., Botvinick, E., Schiller, N. B., Crooks, L., Kaufman, L. and Lipton, M. J. (1984) Imaging by NMR in patients with chronic ischemic heart disease. Circulation 69, 523–531.

Nunally, R. L. and Bottomley, P. A. (1981) 31-P NMR studies of myocardial ischemia and its response to drug therapies. J.Comput.Assist.Tomogr. 5, 296–298.

Ruigrok, T. J. C., Van Echteld, C. J. A., De Kruijff, B., Borst, C. and Miller, F. L. (1983) Protective effect of Nifedipine in myocardial ischemia assessed by 31P-NMR. Eur.Heart J. 4, 109–113.

Wesbey, G., Higgins, C. B., Lanzer, P., Botvinick, E. and Lipton, M. J. (1984) Imaging and characterization of acute myocardial infarction in vivo by gated NMR. Circulation 69, 125–130.

Williams, E. S., Kaplan, J. L., Thatcher, F., Zimmerman, G. and Knoebel, S. B. (1980) Prolongation of proton spin-lattice relaxation times in regionally ischemic tissue from dog hearts. J.Nucl.Med. 21, 449–453.

Flow

Battocletti, J. H., Halback, R. E., Sallescu, S. X. and Sances, A. (1981) NMR blood-flowmeter: theory and history. Med.Phys. 8, 435–443.

Bryant, D. J., Payne, J. A., Firmin, D. N. and Longmore, D. B. (1984) Measurement of flow with NMR imaging using a gradient pulse and phase difference technique. J.Comput.Assist.Tomogr. 8, 588–593.

Crooks, L. and Kaufman, L. (1984) NMR imaging of blood flow. Br.Med.Bull. 40, 167–170.

Dijk, P. (1984) Direct cardiac NMRI of heart wall and blood flow velocity. J.Comput.Assist.Tomogr. 18, 429–437.

George, C. R., Jacobs, G., MacIntyre, W. J., Lorig, R. J., Go, R. T., Nox, Y. and Meany, T. F. (1984) MR signal intensing patterns obtained from continuous and pulsative flow models. Radiology 151, 421–428.

Grant, J. P. and Back, C. (1982) NMR rheotomography: feasibility and clinical potential. Med.Phys. 9, 188–193.

Hemminga, M. A. and Dejager, P. A. (1980) The study of flow by pulsed NMR: II. Measurement of flow velocities using a repetitive method. J.Magn.Reson. 37, 1–16.

Mills, C. M., Brant-Zawadzki, M., Crooks, L. E., Kaufman, L., Sheldon, P., Norman, D., Bank, W. and Newton, T. H. (1983) NMR: Principles of blood flow imaging. AJNR 4, 1161–1166.

Singer, J. R. (1959) Blood flow rates by NMR measurements. Science 130, 1652–1653.

Singer, J. R. (1981) NMR flow imaging. Symposium, Winston-Salem, NC, 1–3 October 1981, pp. 185–190.

Van As, H. and Schaapsma, T. J. (1985) Flow imaging. In 'NMR Tomography'. Eds., Rinck, P. A., Pedersen, S. B. and Mullen, R. N., Georg Thieme Verlag, Stuttgart, Ch. VIII.

Waluch, V. and Bradley, W. G. (1984) NMR even echo rephasing in slow laminar flow. J.Comput.Assist.Tomogr. 8, 594–598.

Webb, W. R., Gamsu, G., Golden, J. A. and Grooks, L. E. (1984) NMR of pulmonary arteriovenous fistula effects of flow. J.Comput.Assist.Tomogr. 8, 155–157.

Miscellaneous

Pavlicek, W., Geisinger, M., Castle, L., Borkowski, G. P., Meany, T. F., Bream, B. L. and Gallagher, J. H. (1983) The effects of NMR on patients with cardiac pacemakers. Radiology 147, 149–153.

Abdominal organs

Liver, gallbladder

Aisen, A. M., Martel, W., Glazer, G. M. and Carson, P. L. (1983) Hepatic imaging: PET, DSA, NMR. Hepatology 3, 1024–1030.

Bernardino, M. E., Small, W., Goldstein, J., Sewell, C. W., Jones, P. J., Gedgandas-McClees, K., Galambos, J. T., Wenger, J. and Casarella, W. J. (1983) Multiple NMR T_2 relaxation values in human liver tissue. AJR 141, 1203–1208.

Borkowski, G. P., Buonocore, E., George, C. R., Go, R. T., O'Donovan, P. B. and Meany, T. F. (1983) NMR imaging in the evaluation of the liver. A preliminary experience. J.Comput.Assist.Tomogr. 7, 768–774.

Cohen, S. M. (1983) Application of NMR to the study of liver, physiology and disease. Hepatology 3, 738–749.

Davis, P. L., Kaufman, L., Crooks, L. E. and Miller, T. R. (1981) Detectability of hepatomas in rat livers by NMR imaging. Invest.Radiol. 16, 354–359.

Doyle, F. H., Pennock, J. M., Banks, L. M., McDonnel, M. J., Bydder, G. M., Steiner, R. E., Young, I. R., Clarke, G. J., Pasmore, T. and Gilderdale, D. J. (1982) NMRI of the liver: initial experience. AJR 138, 193–200.

Hawkes, R. C., Holland, G. N., Moore, W. S., Roebuck, E. J. and Worthington, B. S. (1981) NMR tomography of the normal heart and abdomen. J.Comput.Assist.Tomogr. 5, 605–618.

Hricak, H., Filly, R. A., Margulis, A. R., Moon, K. L., Crooks, L. E. and Kaufman, L. (1983) NMR imaging of the gallbladder. Radiology 147, 481–484.

Jacobs, D. D., Albina, J. E., Gregg Settle, R., Wolf, G. and Rombeau, J. L. (1983) In vitro identification of carbon tetrachloride induced fatty liver infiltration by NMR. Surg.Forum 34, 54–56.

Kressel, H. Y., Axel, L., Glover, G. and Baum, S. (1984) Coronal NMR imaging of the abdomen at 0.5 Tesla. J.Comput.Assist.Tomogr. 8, 29–31.

Lawler, G. A., Pennock, J. M., Steiner, R. E., Jenkins, W. J., Sherlock, S. and Young, I. R. (1983) NMR imaging in liver disease: Wilson disease. J.Comput.Assist.Tomogr. 7, 1–8.

186   Margulis, A. R., Moss, A. A., Crooks, L. E. and Kaufman, L. (1983) NMR in the diagnosis of tumors of the liver. Semin.Roentgenol. 18, 123–126.

Moon, K. L., Hricak, H., Margulis, A. R., Bernhoff, R., Way, L. W., Filly, R. A. and Crooks, L. E. (1983) NMR imaging of gallstones in vitro. Radiology 148, 753–756.

Moss, A. A., Goldberg, H. I., Stark, D. B., Davis, P. L., Margulis, A. R., Kaufman, L. and Crooks, L. E. (1984) Hepatic tumors. NMR and CT appearance. Radiology 150, 141–147.

Newhouse, J. H., Brady, T. J., Gebhardt, M., Burt, C. T., Pykett, I. L., Goldman, M. R., Buonanno, F. S., Kistler, J. P., Hinshaw, W. S. and Pohost, G. M. (1982) NMRI: Preliminary results in the upper extremities of man and the abdomen of small animals (abstract). Radiology 142, 246.

Rödl, W., Lutz, H. and Oppelt, A. (1983) NMR imaging in abdominal and pelvic disease; initial clinical experience in comparison with CT and US. Hepatogastroenterology 30, 37–41.

Runge, V. M., Clanton, J. A., Smith, F. W., Hutchison, J., Mallard, J., Partain, C. L. and James, A. E. (1983) NMR of iron and copper disease states. AJR 141, 943–948.

Smith, F. W., Hutchison, J. M., Mallard, J. R., Johnson, G., Redpath, T. W., Selbie, R. D., Reid, A. and Smith, C. C. (1981) Oesophageal carcinoma demonstrated by whole-body NMR. Br.Med.J. 282, 510–512.

Smith, F. W., Mallard, J. R., Reid, A. and Hutchison, J. M. S. (1981) NMR tomographic imaging in liver disease. Lancet I, 963–966.

Stark, D. D., Bass, N. M., Moss, A. A., Bacon, B. R., McKerrow, J. H., Cann, C. E., Brito, A. and Goldberg, H. I. (1983) NMR imaging of experimentally induced liver disease. Radiology 148, 743–751.

Stark, D. D., Goldberg, H. I., Moss, A. A. and Bass, N. M. (1984) Chronic liver disease: evaluation by NMR. Radiology 150, 149–151.

Pancreas

Smith, F. W., Reid, A., Hutchison, J. M. S., Mallard, J. R. and Path, F. R. C. (1982) NMR imaging of the pancreas. Radiology 142, 667–680.

Stark, D. D., Moss, A. A., Goldberg, H. I., Deveney, C. W. and Way, L. (1983) CT and NMR imaging of pancreatic islet cell tumors. Surgery 94, 1024–1027.

Stark, D. D., Moss, A. A., Goldberg, H. I., Davis, P. L. and Federle, M. P. (1984) MR and CT of the normal and diseased pancreas: a comparative study. Radiology 150, 153–162.

Kidneys, adrenal glands, pelvis

Brasch, R. C., London, D. A., Wesbey, G. E., Tozer, T. N., Nitechi, D. E., Williams, R. D., Doemeny, J., Tuck, L. D. and Lallemand, D. P. (1983) Work in progress: NMR study of a paramagnetic nitroxide contrast agent for enhancement of renal structures in experimental animals. Radiology 147, 773–779.

Choyke, P. L., Kressel, H. Y., Pollack, H. M., Arger, P. M., Axel, L. and Mamourian, A. C. (1984) Focal renal masses: magnetic resonance imaging. Radiology 152, 471–478.

Hricak, H., Crooks, L., Sheldon, P. and Kaufman, L. (1983) NMR imaging of the kidney. Radiology 146, 425–432.

Hricak, H., Higgins, C. B. and Williams, R. D. (1983) NMR imaging in retroperitoneal fibrosis. AJR 141, 35–38.

Hricak, H., Williams, R. D., Moon, K. L., Moss, A. A., Alpers, C., Crooks, L. E. and Kaufman, L. (1983) NMR imaging of the kidney: renal masses. Radiology 147, 765–772.

Hricak, H., Williams, R. D., Spring, D. B., Moon, K. L., Hedgecock, M. W., Warson, R. A. and Crooks, L. E. (1983) Anatomy and pathology of the male pelvis by MRI. AJR 141, 1101–1110.

London, D. A., Davis, P. L., Williams, R. D., Crooks, L. E., Sheldon, P. E. and Gooding, C. A. (1983) NMR imaging of induced renal lesions. Radiology 148, 167–172.

Moon, K. L., Hricak, H., Crooks, L. E., Gooding, C. A., Moss, A. A., Engelstad, B. L. and Kaufman, L. (1983) NMR imaging of the adrenal gland: a preliminary report. Radiology 147, 155–160.

Ruijs, J. H. (1982) NMR case study – diagnosis of Grawitz tumor – recurrence by NMR scan. Medica Mundi 27, 97.

Slutsky, R. A., Andre, M. P., Mattrey, R. F. and Brahme, F. J. (1984) In vitro magnetic relaxation times of the ischaemic and reperfused rabbit kidney. J.Nucl.Med. 25, 38–41.

Smith, F. W., Hutchison, J. M. S., Mallard, J. R., Reid, A., Johnson, G., Redpath, T. W. and Selbie, R. D. (1982) Renal cyst or tumor. Differentiation by whole-body NMRI. Diagn.Imaging 50, 61–65.

Smith, F. W., Reid, A., Mallard, J. R., Hutchison, J. M. S., Power, D. A. and Catto, G. R. D. (1982) NMR tomographic imaging in renal disease. Diagn.Imaging 51, 209–213.

Steyn, J. H. and Smith, F. W. (1982) NMR imaging of the prostate. Br.J.Urol. 54, 726–728.

Thickman, D., Kundel, H. and Biery, D. (1984) Magnetic resonance evaluation of hydronephrosis in the dog. Radiology 152, 113–116.

Chest

Mammae

Bovée, W. M. M. J., Getreuer, K. W., Smidt, J. and Lindeman, J. (1978) NMR and detection of human breast tumors. J.Natl.Cancer.Inst. 61, 53–55.

Davis, P. L., Sheldon, P., Kaufman, L., Crooks, L., Margulis, A. R., Miller, T., Watts, J., Arakawa, M. and Hoeninger, J. (1983) NMR of mammary adenocarcinomas in the rat. Cancer 51, 433–439.

El Yousef, S. J., Alfidi, R. J., Duchesneau, R. H., Hubay, C. A., Haaga, J. R., Bryan, P. J., LiPuma, J. P. and Ament, A. E. (1983) Initial experience with NMR imaging of the human breast. J.Comput.Assist.Tomogr. 7, 215–218.

Medina, D. (1979) NMR studies on human breast dysplasias and neoplasms. J.Natl.Cancer Inst. 54, 813–818.

Ross, R. J., Thompson, J. S., Kim, K. and Bailey, R. A. (1982) NMR imaging and evaluation of human breast tumors: preliminary clinical trials. Radiology 143, 195–205.

Mediastinum and hili

Cohen, A. M., Creviston, S., LiPuma, J. P., Bryan, P. J., Haaga, J. R. and Alfidi, R. J. (1983) NMR evaluation of hilar and mediastinal lymphadenopathy. Radiology 148, 739–742.

Gamsu, G., Stark, D. D., Webb, W. R., Moore, E. H. and Sheldon, P. E. (1984) MRI of benign mediastinal masses. Radiology 151, 709–713.

Steiner, R. E. (1984) NMR imaging of the heart and mediastinum. Br.Med.Bull. 40, 191–194.

Webb, W. R., Gamsu, G. and Crooks, L. E. (1984) Multisection sagittal and coronal MRI of the mediastinum and hila. Radiology 150, 475–478.

Webb, W. R., Gamsu, G., Stark, D. D. and Moore, E. H. (1984) Magnetic resonance imaging of the normal and abnormal pulmonary hila. Radiology 152, 89–94.

Thoracic diseases

Brasch, R. C., Gooding, C. A., Lallemand, D. P. and Wesbey, G. E. (1984) MRI of the thorax in childhood. Radiology 150, 463–467.

Frank, J. A., Feiler, M. A., House, W. V., Lauterbur, P. C. and Jacobson, M. J. (1976) Measurement of proton NMR longitudinal relaxation time and water content in infarcted canine myocardium and induced pulmonary injury. Clin.Res. 24, 217A.

Gamsu, G., Webb, W. R., Sheldon, P., Kaufman, L., Crooks, L. E., Binnberg, F. A., Goodman, P., Hinchcliffe, W. A. and Hedgecock, M. (1983) NMR imaging of the thorax. Radiology 147, 473–480.

Kundel, H. L., Kressel, H. Y. and Epstein, D. (1983) The potential role of NMR imaging in thoracic disease. Radiol.Clin.N.Am. 21, 801–808.

Ross, J. S., O'Donovan, P. B., Novoa, R., Mehta, A., Buonocore, E., McIntyre, W. J., Golish, W. A. and Ahmed, M. (1984) Magnetic resonance of the chest: initial experience with imaging and in vivo T_1 and T_2 calculations. Radiology 152, 95–101.

Runge, V. M., Clanton, J. A., Partain, C. L. and James, A. E. (1984) Respiratory gating in MRI at 0.5 T. Radiology 151, 521–523.

Webb, W. R., Gamsu, G., Golden, J. A. and Crooks, L. E. (1984) NMR of pulmonary arteriovenous fistula: effects of flow. J.Comput.Assist.Tomogr. 8, 155–157.

Gynaecology and obstetrics

Bryan, P. J., Butler, H. E., LiPuma, J. P., Haaga, J. R., El Yousef, S. J., Resnick, M. I., Cohen, A. M., Malviya, V. K., Nelson, A. D., Clampitt, M., Alfidi, B., Cohen, J. and Morrison, S. C. (1983) NMR scanning of the pelvis: initial experience with a 0.3 T system. AJR 141, 1111–1118.

Foster, M. A., Knight, C. H., Rimmington, J.E. and Mallard, J. R. (1983) Fetal imaging by NMR: a study in goats. Radiology 149, 193–195.

Hricak, H., Alpers, C., Crooks, L. E. and Sheldon, P. E. (1983) Anatomy and pathology of the female pelvis by MRI. AJR 141, 1119–1128.

Johnson, I. R., Symonds, E. M., Kean, D. M., Johnson, J., Gyngell, M. and Hawkes, R. C. (1984) Imaging of ovarian tumors by NMR. Br.J.Obstet.Gynaecol. 91, 260–264.

Langner, K., Schmidt, S., Dudenhau, J. W., Saling, E., Friedbur, H., Hopfel, D. and Helledie, N. (1984) Measurement of fetal pH in the guinea pig by NMR. Lancet I, 1361.

Mann, W. J., Mendonça-Dias, M. H., Lauterbur, P. C., Klimek, R., Stone, M. L.,   189
Bernardo, M. L. Jr., Chumas, J. C., Heidelberger, R., Acuff, V. and Taylor, A.
(1984) Preliminary in vitro studies of NMR spin lattice relaxation times and three
dimensional NMRI in gynaecologic oncology. Am.J.Obstet.Gynaecol. 148, 91–95.
Smith, F. W. and McLennan, R. S. (1984) NMR imaging in human pregnancy: a
preliminary study. Magn.Reson.Imaging 2, 57–64.
Smith, F. W., Adam, A. H. and Philips, W. D. P. (1983) NMR imaging in pregnancy.
Lancet I, 61–62.
Younkin, D. P., Leonard, J. C., Delivori, M., Subraman, H. and Chance, B. (1983)
Unique features of human newborn cortical metabolism measured with ^{31}P-NMR.
Ann.Neurol. 14, 355.

Skeleton, orthopedic surgical applications

Berquist, T. H. (1984) Preliminary experience in orthopedic radiology. Magn.Re-
son.Imaging 2, 41–52.
Brady, T. J., Gebhardt, M. C., Pykett, I. L., Buonanno, F. S., Newhouse, J. H., Burt, C.
T., Smith, R. J., Mankin, H. J., Kistler, J. P., Goldman, M. R., Hinshaw, W. S. and
Pohost, G. M. (1982) NMRI of forearms in healthy volunteers and patients with
giant cell tumor of bone. Radiology 144, 549–552.
Brady, T. J., Rosen, B. R., Pykett, I. L., McGuire, M. H., Mankin, H. J. and Rosenthal,
D. I. (1983) NMR imaging of leg tumors. Radiology 149, 181–187.
Cherryman, G.R. and Smith, F. W. (1984) NMR scanning for skeletal tumours. Lancet
23 June, 1403–1404.
Cohen, M. D., Klatte, E. C., Baehner, R., Smith, J. A., Martin-Simmerman, P., Carr,
B. E., Provisor, A. J., Weetman, R. M., Coates, T., Siddiqui, A., Weisman, S. J.,
Berkow, R., McKenna, S. and McGuire W. A. (1984) MRI of bone marrow disease
in children. Radiology 151, 715–718.
Hinshaw, W. S., Andrew, E. R., Bottomley, P. A., Holland, G. N., Moore, W. S. and
Worthington, B. S. (1979) An in vivo study of the forearm and hand by thin section
NMR imaging. Br.J.Radiol. 52, 36–43.
Hull, R. G., Rennie, J. A. N., Eastmond, C. J., Hutchison, J. M. S. and Smith, F. W.
(1984) NMR tomographic imaging for popliteal cysts in rheumatoid arthritis.
Ann.Rheum.Dis. 43, 56–59.
Kean, C. M., Worthington, B. S., Preston, B. J., Roebuck, E. J., McKim-Thomas, H.,
Hawkes, R. C., Holland, G. M. and Moore, W. S. (1983) NMR of the knee.
Br.J.Radiol. 56, 355–364.
Moon, K. L., Genant, H. K., Helms, C. A., Chafetz, N. I., Crooks, L. E. and Kaufman,
L. (1983) Musculo skeletal applications of NMR. Radiology 147, 161–171.
Newhouse, J. H., Brady, T. J., Gebhardt, M., Burt, C. T., Pykett, I. L., Goldman, M. R.,
Buonanno, F. S., Kistler, J. P., Hinshaw, W. S. and Pohost, G. M. (1982) NMRI:
Preliminary results in the upper extremities of man and the abdomen of small ani-
mals (abstract). Radiology 142, 246.
Sepponen, R. E., Sipponen, J. T. and Tantta, J. I. (1984) A method for chemical shift
imaging: demonstration of bone marrow involvement with proton chemical shift
imaging. J.Comput.Assist.Tomogr. 8, 585–587.

Subject index